# CORONARY HEART DISEASE

## From Diagnosis to Treatment

**Third Edition**

**BARRY M. COHEN, M.D.**

Addicus Books
Omaha, Nebraska

**An Addicus Nonfiction Book**

ISBN: 978-1-943886-85-2

Interior and cover design by Jack Kusler

This book is not intended to be a substitute for a physician, nor do the authors intend to give advice contrary to that of an attending physician.

**Library of Congress Cataloging-in-Publication Data**
Names: Cohen, Barry M., author.
Title: Coronary heart disease: from diagnosis to treatment/ Barry M. Cohen, M.D.
Description: Third edition. | Omaha, Nebraska: Addicus Books, [2019] | Includes index.
Identifiers: LCCN 2018059484 (print) | LCCN 2018059736 (ebook) | ISBN 9781950091003 (pdf) | ISBN 9781950091027 (kdl) | ISBN 9781950091010 (epub) | ISBN 9781943886852 (alk. paper)
Subjects: LCSH: Coronary heart disease—Popular works.
Classification: LCC RC685.C6 (ebook) | LCC RC685.C6 C58 2019 (print) | DDC 616.1/23—dc23
LC record available at https://lccn.loc.gov/2018059484

Addicus Books, Inc.
P.O. Box 45327
Omaha, Nebraska 68145
www.AddicusBooks.com

Printed in the United States of America
10 9 8 7 6 5 4 3 2 1

*To my wife Jill and our children*
*Sara, Brett, and Chloe*

# CONTENTS

*The physician should not treat the disease
but the patient who is suffering from it.*
—Maimonides,
philosopher 1135–1204

# ACKNOWLEDGMENTS

I am deeply grateful for the assistance and insights from colleagues, friends, and family who helped make this book possible. From the Morristown and Overlook Medical Centers' Gagnon Cardiovascular Institute in New Jersey, I would like to thank Dr. Linda Gillam and my colleagues in cardiology and cardiac surgery as well as the team from the Chambers Center for Well Being. They were all invaluable resources. Kathy Cohen, R.D., of the Toronto Western Hospital was exceptionally helpful sharing her perspectives and expertise in nutrition.

I am deeply indebted to Dr. Valentin Fuster and my former professors and mentors from Mount Sinai Medical Center in New York, Dr. Maurice Buchbinder and the faculty of the University of California San Diego Medical Center, as well as the Jewish General Hospital–McGill University in Montreal, and the University of Sherbrooke. I acknowledge Drs. Irwin Labin, Ken Aaron, Danny Bercovitch, Mr. Herbert Bernard, and the late Drs. Seymour Cohen and Harold Frank.

I would also like to thank my publisher, Rod Colvin of Addicus Books, for his outstanding editing skills and for his clear vision for this book. Without Rod, this project would not be a reality. I also thank Jack Kusler for his original illustrations and design work.

I am deeply appreciative of my parents, Elaine and Gerry Cohen, for their love, guidance, and encouragement throughout my studies and medical career. My parents have also been role models to me. Their more than seventy years of marriage is a testament to their heart-healthy lifestyle. I also thank my wife's parents, Ellen and Sam Weinstock, for their assistance and advice.

I'd like to thank my many patients and their families who have given me a great sense of professional and personal fulfillment as well as a heightened commitment to humanity each and every day.

We are all indebted to Nobel laureates Sir Frederick Grant Banting and John Macleod, and to Charles Best, for their discovery of insulin in 1921 at the University of Toronto. Their discovery is one of the most dramatic events in the history of medicine.

Finally, I am most grateful to my wonderful wife Jill, and our amazing children, Sara, Brett, and Chloe, for their love, encouragement, and endless support.

—Barry M. Cohen, M.D.

# INTRODUCTION

Despite the many advances in the diagnosis and treatment of coronary heart disease, this condition remains the most common cause of death and reduced quality of life for men and women. Perhaps you have coronary heart disease, but even if you don't, you almost certainly know someone who does.

In this new edition of *Coronary Heart Disease: From Diagnosis to Treatment,* cardiologist Barry Cohen, M.D. provides an easy-to-understand resource for those who want to learn more about coronary heart disease—its causes and ways to prevent it.

Dr. Cohen is a master clinician and expert in treating coronary heart disease. From him you will learn the risk factors for coronary heart disease along with state-of-the-art tools used for diagnosis and treatment. You will learn about the methods to reopen partially or completely blocked arteries—medications, stenting, and bypass surgery. You will also gain an understanding of medications that are commonly used to modify risk factors, control symptoms, and reduce the likelihood of a heart attack. And, importantly, you will learn about the important coronary heart disease differences between men and women.

This is a must read for anyone who would like to reduce their likelihood of getting coronary heart disease and for those who are living with it. Share the information you learn here with those you love and use it to improve communications with your own health care team. The overarching goal is to help you live a healthier life.

—Linda D. Gillam, M.D., M.P.H.
Dorothy and Lloyd Huck Chair
Department of Cardiovascular Medicine
Morristown Medical Center

# 1 CORONARY HEART DISEASE: AN OVERVIEW

When a doctor tells you that you have coronary heart disease, it can be worrisome and confusing. You undoubtedly have questions: What is coronary heart disease? Why did I get it? Do I need medication? Will I need surgery? Do I need to change my lifestyle? Hopefully, this book will answer these questions and many more.

## What Is Coronary Heart Disease?

*Coronary heart disease (CHD),* also called *ischemic heart disease,* is a form of heart disease that's caused by narrowing of the coronary arteries that feed the heart. If you or someone you love has been diagnosed with CHD, it may help to know that you are not alone.

### How Many People Have CHD?

CHD is the most common form of heart disease, affecting at least 16 million Americans. It is the single largest killer of both men and women in the United States, responsible for nearly a half million deaths each year, or about one out of every five deaths. CHD causes the vast majority of heart attacks *(myocardial infarctions).* Every forty seconds, someone in the United States suffers a coronary event, and every minute one of us will die from one. The American Heart Association estimates that this year alone, more than a million

Americans will suffer from a new or recurring coronary event, and nearly 40 percent of those will die from it.

Coronary heart disease isn't just an American problem. It is also very common in Europe and other Westernized countries. Diseases of the heart and circulation, such as heart attacks and strokes, kill more people worldwide than any other cause. The World Health Organization estimates that as many as 30 percent of all deaths worldwide are caused by heart and circulation diseases such as CHD.

### Reducing Risk

There is much you can do to reduce your risk of having a heart attack or dying from CHD. Sometimes just changing your lifestyle—following a heart-healthy diet, exercising regularly, and reducing the stress in your life—can prevent a heart attack or even reverse the narrowing in your arteries.

There are a number of medications—and new ones being developed every day—that can help lower your heart attack risk. Surgical procedures to open blocked arteries, or bypass surgery, can help compensate for blockages in your arteries and help keep your heart supplied with the blood it needs.

By educating yourself about treatment options with books such as this one and by working closely with your doctor, you can choose the treatments that will best enable you to live a long and healthy life.

## The Circulatory System

The first step in taking charge of your CHD is to learn all you can about the disease. To understand what CHD is and how it affects your heart, you need to understand a little about your heart and how it works.

The *circulatory system* is made up of the heart, the lungs, and blood vessels called *arteries* and *veins*. This system carries blood, food, and oxygen to every cell in the

## Exterior of the Heart

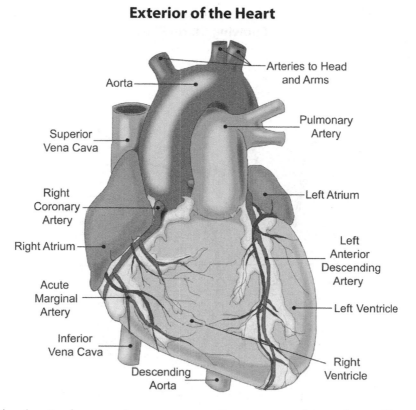

body. It also carries waste products away from the cells and out of the body. Arteries carry blood enriched with oxygen and nutrients away from the heart to the cells in the body. Veins carry blood loaded with waste products from the cells back to the heart.

Between the blood vessels, *capillaries*—thinner than a strand of hair—connect the smallest arteries with the smallest veins. The walls of these tiny capillaries allow waste products from the cells to pass into the capillaries. This enables the blood to carry waste from the cells to be removed by the kidneys, liver, and lungs.

3

## Interior of the Heart
### Showing Blood Flow

Superior Vena Cava

Aorta

Pulmonary Artery

to Lungs

to Lungs

Pulmonary Veins

from Lungs

Left Atrium

Right Atrium

Left Ventricle

Right Ventricle

Inferior Vena Cava

Ventricular Septum

### *The Heart: An Amazing Pump*

The heart is the pump that keeps the blood flowing around and around in an endless circle throughout the body. The heart is a hollow muscle that weighs less than a pound and is about the size of a man's fist. Despite its small size, this amazing organ beats an average of 100,000 times a day, pumping about 2,000 gallons of blood every day. By the time you are age seventy, your heart will have beaten more than 2.5 billion times.

Located in the center of the chest and protected by the breastbone and rib cage, the heart is actually a double

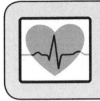

**Heart Notes**

If the body's blood vessels were laid end to end, they'd cover about 60,000 miles—more than twice the circumference of the earth!

pump that's divided into two upper chambers and two lower ones. A wall of tissue separates the left and right sides of the heart. The top chambers *(atria)* and lower chambers *(ventricles)* are connected by valves that act like one-way doors. These valves make sure blood flows only in one direction. In the heart, the blood is pumped from the left and right atria to the left and right ventricles. The right side of the heart sends blood to the lungs. The left side of the heart pumps blood out to the cells in the body.

## Coronary Arteries

Just like other muscles in the body, the heart needs its own supply of blood and oxygen to work properly. Even though the heart pumps blood through its chambers, the heart itself receives little nourishment from this blood. A separate set of arteries that branch off the aorta (the main artery that receives blood from the left ventricle) provide the heart's blood supply. These are called *coronary arteries.* The coronary arteries encircle the top and sides of the heart, bringing it oxygen-rich blood. The two major coronary arteries are the *left coronary artery* and the *right coronary artery.* These vessels divide into many smaller coronary arteries that feed the heart.

## What Causes Coronary Heart Disease?

The walls of the arteries that provide blood to the heart have a smooth, flexible surface. However, over many years, these walls can become progressively irritated and damaged. The damage may result from substances such as fats, cholesterol, calcium, cellular debris, and platelets—the tiny cells responsible for blood

5

## Atherosclerosis Formation

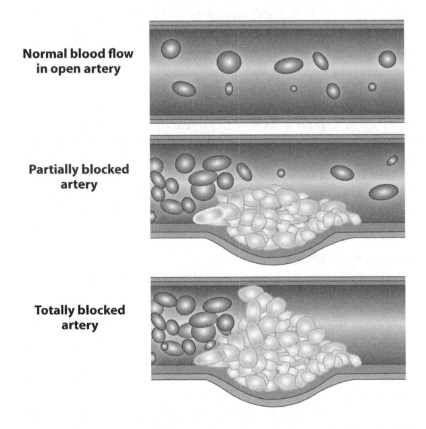

Normal blood flow
in open artery

Partially blocked
artery

Totally blocked
artery

Atherosclerosis occurs when plaque deposits block the flow of blood in arteries.

clotting. When the artery walls become damaged, these substances can stick to them; coronary heart disease occurs when the arteries become narrowed and clogged.

### Buildup of Plaque

This buildup of substances inside the artery walls is a process called *atherosclerosis,* which produces a substance known as *plaque.* As it accumulates, plaque acts a lot like the dirt and minerals that build up inside your home's plumbing. As the buildup becomes thicker, the flow through the pipes becomes clogged and may eventually stop.

Similarly, when your heart doesn't get enough oxygen, due to narrowed arteries, you may feel chest pressure or pain called *angina*. If the blood supply to part of the heart is completely cut off, the result is often a heart attack.

Everyone has a certain amount of atherosclerosis as they age. For many of us, atherosclerosis begins in childhood. Some people have a rapid increase in the buildup of atherosclerotic plaque after age thirty. For others, plaque buildup doesn't become a problem until they're in their fifties or sixties. You may hear the word *arteriosclerosis* being used interchangeably with atherosclerosis. The difference in the two words is technical. Arteriosclerosis refers to hardening of the arteries.

### Why Atherosclerosis Develops

It's not fully understood why atherosclerosis occurs, but there are several theories. Some medical experts believe that the atherosclerotic buildup in the inner layers of the arteries may be caused by several conditions, including:

- elevated levels of LDL cholesterol (low-density lipoprotein) and triglycerides (a type of blood fat in the blood)
- low levels of HDL cholesterol (high-density lipoprotein)
- stress
- high blood pressure
- smoking
- high blood sugar levels (diabetes)
- sedentary lifestyle
- inflammation in the artery walls
- genetics

7

It's likely that more than one process is involved in the buildup of plaque. Many researchers believe that when excess fats combine, they become trapped in the artery walls. Then, any injury to the artery wall, such as damage caused by smoking, can cause more damage. Plaque grows, causing narrowing of arteries or causing blood clots to form. Advanced plaque consists of cell debris, calcium, smooth muscle cells, fatty deposits, connective tissue, and foam cells, which are white blood cells that have digested fat.

Cells containing plaque can be easily damaged. This can lead to blood clots forming on the outside of the plaque. Small clots can further damage other layers of the blood vessel wall and stimulate more plaque growth. Larger blood clots can partially or totally block the artery.

In addition to blocking blood flow, plaque can hinder the arteries' ability to dilate and contract. In order to respond to the body's ever-changing need for blood, the arteries need to be strong and elastic. For instance, when you exercise, your body needs more blood. The heart responds by pumping faster, and the arteries respond by expanding to accommodate the increased volume of blood coming from the heart. As the artery becomes narrowed and hard, that elasticity is lost. Arteries that have atherosclerotic plaque are more apt to spasm (temporarily narrow), causing even less blood to flow to the heart and possibly causing chest pain or a heart attack.

### Inflammation and High Blood Pressure

Other conditions that may also damage the arteries include inflammation and high blood pressure. *Inflammation* refers to the body's natural defense to foreign invaders such as bacteria, toxins, or viruses. The tissues become inflamed.

*High blood pressure* occurs when the pressure of blood flowing through arteries is too high. Arteries are strong and elastic, enabling them to withstand pressure as the heart pumps; however, when blood pressure is

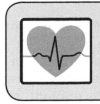

**Heart Notes**

Arteries are strong and elastic, making them able to withstand pressure as the heart pumps. Veins have valves to help blood return to the heart.

too high, there is a chance that the extra pressure could weaken an artery. And, if your arteries are narrowed, there is a greater risk that they could become blocked. High blood pressure can lead to a heart attack, stroke, and other heart ailments.

## Metabolic Syndrome and CHD

One of the conditions associated with the development of coronary heart disease is *metabolic syndrome.* Not an actual disease itself, metabolic syndrome is a cluster of disorders. According to current guidelines from the American Heart Association and the National Cholesterol Education Program, you have metabolic syndrome if you have three or more of the following conditions:

- high-fasting blood sugar levels (insulin resistance)
- high blood pressure
- low HDL cholesterol
- high triglycerides
- abdominal obesity—a waist circumference of forty inches or more in men, thirty-five inches or more in women.

Each of these disorders is associated with cardiovascular disease, stroke, and diabetes and the collective effect of metabolic syndrome significantly increases the risk of death from these diseases. One study reports that those with metabolic syndrome are 3.5 times more likely to die of a heart-related problem and 5 times as likely to develop type 2 diabetes.

## High Blood Sugars

The core disorder of metabolic syndrome is insulin resistance, which explains why the condition is sometimes referred to as *insulin resistance syndrome*. Insulin is a hormone that controls the amount of sugar (glucose) in your bloodstream. When your body doesn't make enough insulin or use insulin efficiently, the result is higher levels of glucose in your blood. The high blood sugars increase the risk for CHD. The high glucose levels can damage blood vessels and nerves that control the heart. Individuals with diabetes tend to develop heart disease at a younger age.

## How Common Is Metabolic Syndrome?

Metabolic syndrome is becoming increasingly common. It's estimated that 34 percent of the American population has metabolic syndrome; 85 percent with type 2 diabetes have it. Two other key actors that cause metabolic syndrome—obesity and physical inactivity—are related to lifestyle. Other factors include aging, genetic predisposition, hormonal imbalance, and a history of diabetes.

# 2 RISK FACTORS FOR CORONARY HEART DISEASE

Perhaps you've wondered why you developed coronary heart disease. It's not fully known why some people develop CHD while others do not. We do know that certain factors—traits or lifestyle habits—increase your chance of having a heart attack or stroke. The more risk factors you have, the higher the likelihood that you'll have a buildup of atherosclerotic plaque. That's why it's important to understand and control the risk factors for CHD.

According to the National Heart, Lung, and Blood Institute of the National Institutes of Health, having multiple risk factors for CHD doesn't just add to your risk, it multiplies it. If, for instance, you're a smoker who has high blood pressure and high blood cholesterol, your risk for CHD is eight times greater than someone with no risk factors.

Most risk factors for CHD can be changed. Others, such as increasing age, family history, your race or gender, obviously, cannot.

## Risk Factors You Can't Control

### Increasing Age

The older you are, the greater your risk for CHD, heart attack, and stroke. Four out of five people who die from CHD are sixty-five or older. If you're a man forty-five years or older, you're at increased risk for heart attack or stroke. If you're a woman fifty-five years or older, or

11

you're past menopause, or you have had your ovaries removed at a young age, you are at increased risk. The aging process itself is partly to blame. As we age, the connective tissues in our artery walls naturally become less flexible. As mentioned earlier, this is called arteriosclerosis, or "hardening of the arteries." This loss of flexibility in the arteries can cause blood pressure to increase, which can damage arteries and lead to the buildup of plaque. Rising blood pressure and hardened arteries can also make the heart work harder, which can cause the heart muscle to thicken and stiffen. When this occurs, the heart cannot function efficiently.

### Family History of Heart Disease

If members of your family suffered from heart disease, you have a greater risk for CHD, heart attack, and stroke. You have even greater risk if your father or brother had a heart attack before age fifty-five or if your mother or sister had one before age sixty-five. You're also at increased risk if you have a relative who had a stroke.

Some people inherit genes that make them susceptible to the underlying causes of CHD such as diabetes, obesity, high blood cholesterol, or high blood pressure. For instance, diabetes or high blood pressure tends to run in some families. Other people may inherit risk factors such as *familial hypercholesterolemia,* a genetic disorder that causes excessively high LDL or "bad" blood cholesterol. For others, family lifestyle factors such as smoking, overeating, eating high-fat or processed foods, and not exercising may contribute to increased risk.

If you already have CHD, you're at increased risk for heart attack or stroke. If you've already had a heart attack or stroke, you are at risk for having a second one.

## Race

Some ethnic groups are at greater risk for CHD, heart attacks, and stroke. African Americans have higher rates of high blood pressure, a major risk factor for CHD. Mexican Americans, Native Americans, native Hawaiians, and some Asian Americans also have a higher risk for heart disease. Heart experts suspect higher risk among people in these groups may be related, in part, to their increased rates of obesity, diabetes, and smoking. Being economically disadvantaged or lacking access to good health care may also play a part in higher rates of heart disease and poorer prognosis among some groups.

In Japan, the incidence of CHD is lower than in Western countries, yet when Japanese immigrate to North America, their CHD risk climbs, though not as high as other Americans. This suggests that genetics, race, and environment all play a role in CHD.

## Male Gender

Men have a greater chance of having a heart attack and having one earlier than women. Although this may be due to hormonal differences between men and women, men's rate of heart disease is greater even when compared to postmenopausal women who have lost their gender protection against heart attack.

# Risk Factors You Can Control

## High Blood Cholesterol

Cholesterol is a waxy, fatlike substance that's found in every cell in the body. It's a necessary substance that helps digest fats, strengthens cell linings, and makes up part of some types of hormones and vitamins. However, too much cholesterol can be bad for you, causing artery-clogging plaque.

**Major CHD Risk Factors**

- Increasing age
- Family history of heart disease
- Race
- Male gender
- Personal history of heart disease

- High blood cholesterol
- Smoking
- High blood pressure
- Being overweight
- Physical inactivity
- Diabetes

**Contributing CHD Risk Factors**

- Stress
- Elevated homocysteine levels
- Hormonal factors

- Birth control pills
- Excessive alcohol use

Having high blood cholesterol is one of the most important risk factors for CHD and subsequent heart attacks and strokes. However, risk depends on the type of cholesterol you have. The higher your level of *LDL cholesterol (low-density lipoprotein)*—"bad" cholesterol—the greater your risk. When you have too much LDL cholesterol in your blood, the excess builds up on the walls of the coronary arteries. The opposite is true for "good" cholesterol, *HDL cholesterol (high-density lipoprotein):* having high HDL cholesterol protects against CHD; having low HDL cholesterol is a CHD risk factor.

You get cholesterol in two ways: from the liver and from foods you eat. The liver produces all the cholesterol your body needs. But, many of the foods we eat, such as egg yolks, meats, poultry, and whole dairy products, contain cholesterol. Eating too many of these foods can cause high blood cholesterol. Because high blood cholesterol is such a major risk factor, we'll talk more about it in chapter 3.

## Smoking

The American Heart Association calls smoking "the single most preventable cause of death in the United States." Thirty percent of all deaths from CHD in the United States are caused by smoking. In fact, smokers' risk of heart attack is double that of nonsmokers. Smokers who have heart attacks are twice as likely to die and die suddenly (within an hour) than nonsmokers. If you smoke and have other CHD risk factors, you significantly multiply your risk. For those with advanced atherosclerosis, smoking is especially dangerous.

According to a number of studies, including the famous Framingham Heart Study, smoking is a powerful risk factor for CHD and heart attack. Smoking or being exposed to secondhand smoke can cause the following:

- Blood pressure, heart rate, and the amount of blood pumped by the heart temporarily rise, which causes the heart to work harder.
- Arteries in the legs and arms constrict (narrow).
- Delicate tissues inside the arteries become damaged and are more subject to the buildup of artery-clogging plaque.
- Blood supply to the heart, especially in the tiny vessels supplying the heart muscle, decreases.
- Platelets, the clotting agents in blood, become stickier and tend to clump together, so the blood becomes thicker and clotting time is reduced.
- Plaques that are already built up in the arteries can become destabilized. This promotes rupture (cracks in the inner walls of a blood vessel) and the formation of blood clots inside a blood vessel or chamber of the heart.
- "Bad" LDL cholesterol levels increase, and "good" HDL cholesterol levels decrease.

## High Blood Pressure (HBP)

*Blood pressure* refers to the force of blood pumping from the heart. Blood pressure is expressed as two numbers—for example: 120/70. In such a reading, the top number is called the *systolic blood pressure;* it refers to the pressure when the heart pumps blood into the arteries and out into the body.

The bottom number is called the *diastolic blood pressure.* It refers to the pressure in the arteries when the heart rests between beats as the heart fills with blood and receives oxygen. For a normal blood pressure, the top number should be between 90 and 120. The bottom number should be between 60 and 80. The higher your blood pressure, the greater your risk for CHD, heart attack, and other health problems.

When your blood pressure is too high, your heart must work harder. Over time, this can cause the heart muscle to become larger and thicker and may ultimately weaken the heart, making it unable to meet the body's need for blood and oxygen. High blood pressure damages the arteries and *arterioles* (small arteries), scarring them and making them hard and less elastic. It also speeds up the buildup of atherosclerotic plaque and may lead to heart attacks.

As arteries become narrower, clots are more likely to form and block the blood supply completely. If you have high blood pressure and other CHD risk factors such as obesity, smoking, diabetes, or high blood cholesterol, your risk multiplies. High blood pressure is also associated with stroke, kidney failure, and serious eye damage.

## Being Overweight

Being overweight increases your risk for CHD and heart attack as well as for a number of other health problems. If you carry your excess weight around your waist (often refered to as an "apple shape"), with a waist

## Blood Pressure Categories

| Blood Pressure Category | Systolic (Upper Number) | | Diastolic (Lower Number) |
|---|---|---|---|
| Normal | Less than 120 | and | Less than 80 |
| Elevated | 120 – 129 | and | Less than 80 |
| High Blood Pressure (Hypertension) Stage 1 | 130 – 139 | or | 80 – 89 |
| High Blood Pressure (Hypertension) Stage 2 | 140 or Higher | or | 90 or higher |
| Hypertensive Crisis (Consult your doctor immediately) | Higher than 180 | and/or | 90 – 99 |

*Source: American Heart Association*

circumference of forty inches or more for men. thirty-five inches or more for women, your heart disease risk is even higher. Being overweight:

- forces the heart to work harder
- raises blood pressure
- increases blood cholesterol and triglycerides
- lowers "good" HDL blood cholesterol
- increases the risk for developing diabetes, a risk factor for CHD

### Physical Inactivity

If you're a couch potato, you're at risk for heart disease or heart attack. The risk may be as high as six times that of those who are active. If you don't exercise and you overeat, you may be putting yourself at even greater risk for high blood pressure, high blood cholesterol, and type 2 diabetes.

### Diabetes

Diabetes is a major risk factor for CHD. Diabetes is a chronic condition caused by abnormally high levels of sugar (glucose) in the blood. Insulin produced by the

17

pancreas lowers blood glucose. Diabetes occurs when there is either insufficient production of insulin or the body is unable to use insulin efficiently.

There are two types of diabetes. Type 1 diabetes is the result of the body not producing enough insulin. Type 2 diabetes occurs when cells do not properly respond to the insulin that is produced. The body needs insulin in order to convert sugars into energy for body tissues. Without the proper insulin function, the body has increased levels of sugars in the bloodstream.

Over time, these excess sugars can damage blood vessels and nerves. The damage to vessels makes it easier for blockages to develop. Also, patients with diabetes often have higher cholesterol levels, which increase the possibility of blockages in the coronary arteries.

Two-thirds of people with diabetes die from some form of heart disease. Even when your diabetes is treated and you have blood glucose levels under control, you still have an increased risk for heart disease and stroke. One reason for this may be that diabetes also affects blood cholesterol and triglyceride levels that contribute to CHD. In addition, people with diabetes often have high blood pressure.

## Other Risk Factors

The following risk factors are associated with CHD and heart attack, but additional research needs to be done to find out exactly how, and how much, they contribute to the CHD/ heart attack equation.

### Stress

All of us have stress in our lives and everyone reacts to stress differently. Some people are calm most of the time. Stressful events don't seem to faze them much. Others have a "shorter fuse" and tend to overreact to the smallest stresses. Although heart experts aren't all in agreement about the correlation between heart disease

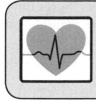 According to the American Heart Association, 50 percent of Americans are at risk for major health problems because of high blood pressure.

and how we react to stress, a growing body of evidence suggests that those who react more negatively to stress may be at greater risk for heart problems.

A six-year study conducted at the University of North Carolina at Chapel Hill found those who were prone to anger were three times more likely to have a heart attack or sudden cardiac death than those who weren't anger-prone. Researchers from Johns Hopkins Hospital reported similar results. They found that people who reacted to stress in a hot-tempered manner were nineteen times more likely to suffer reduced blood flow to the heart, and their coronary arteries and other blood vessels stayed constricted for an abnormally long period of time.

We don't know if stress is an independent risk factor for CHD or if it simply affects other risk factors such as high blood pressure. We do know that stress may cause a person to adopt unhealthful behaviors such as overeating or cigarette smoking, both of which can contribute to heart disease.

### Obstructive Sleep Apnea

*Obstructive sleep apnea (OSA)* is a common health condition in which a person commonly snores and stops breathing briefly in between breaths. This causes drops in oxygen levels. These episodes wake the sleeper as he or she gasps for air. This not only causes sleep disruption, but is also associated with high blood pressure, irregular heartbeats, stroke, and heart failure.

One in five Americans has at least mild sleep apnea. It affects more men than women. The most common type of sleep apnea is caused by body weight on the chest

19

and neck causing the interruption in air flow. Screening for sleep apnea can be performed at a sleep center in a hospital or possibly in your home. Talk to your doctor.

### Elevated Homocysteine Levels

*Homocysteine* is a protein-building substance the body uses for tissue growth. It is acquired mostly by eating meats. In some people, homocysteine clears out of the system, but for others it builds up and increases the risk of cardiovascular disease.

Researchers have speculated that elevated levels of homocysteine may be a cause of atherosclerosis. Research now confirms that elevated levels of homocysteine are associated with CHD. One theory suggests that high levels causes blood vessel walls to narrow. Homocysteine may also cause the development of blood clots.

### Hormonal Factors

Sex hormones affect one's risk for CHD and heart attacks. Female hormones tend to raise "good" HDL cholesterol and reduce "bad" LDL cholesterol. In contrast, male hormones do just the opposite. It's well known that men suffer more heart attacks than women, and men suffer them about ten years earlier than women.

*Female sex hormones.* A number of studies suggest that after menopause, a woman's loss of natural estrogen puts her at higher risk for CHD and heart attack. Women who undergo surgical menopause by the removal of the ovaries and who do not take replacement hormones have a dramatic rise in heart attack risk (similar to men's risk).

*Male sex hormones.* Millions of men take testosterone replacement therapy in an effort to make them feel younger and more energetic as they age. However, there is debate in the medical community as to whether testosterone supplements are beneficial or harmful. In one study, men who took the supplements showed lowered risk of heart disease. However, another study showed potential adverse effects such as heart attacks, heart failure, stroke, personality changes, and infertility.

Some experts say that men should not start testosterone replacement therapy for at least six months after they have had any of the following: heart attack, stent placement for a blocked artery, bypass surgery, heart failure, or stroke.

### Use of Birth Control Pills

Early forms of birth control pills often contained high doses of estrogen. These contraceptives were associated with an increased risk for heart attack and stroke, especially among older women who smoked cigarettes. Newer forms of birth control pills are generally safe—they contain less estrogen and seem to have a lower risk of cardiac problems. However, women over age thirty-five who smoke heavily and take birth control pills are at higher risk for developing blood clots in the legs or lungs.

Women who have used birth control pills in the past are not at increased risk for heart attack later in life.

### Excessive Alcohol Use

Drinking excessively increases the risk for heart disease. Excessive refers to more than one drink per day for women and more than two drinks per day for men. Drinking has been associated with high blood pressure, irregular heartbeats, and high triglycerides. Excessive drinking can also cause heart failure, a condition in which the heart is unable to pump enough blood efficiently. Alcohol consumption also contributes to obesity, another major CHD risk factor.

# 3 UNDERSTANDING CHOLESTEROL

Numerous research studies have established that abnormalities in cholesterol, particularly high LDL ("bad") cholesterol and low HDL ("good") cholesterol, play a major role in the development of CHD and heart attacks. Cholesterol is one of the major components of artery-clogging plaque, so it's important to understand cholesterol's relationship to heart disease.

As mentioned in chapter 2, cholesterol, a waxy, fat-like substance, is necessary for life—it helps in the building of cell structure. However, the body needs only a small amount of cholesterol. The liver produces about 1,000 milligrams of cholesterol every day, or about 80 percent of your blood cholesterol. That's all the cholesterol your body really needs.

But, we also get cholesterol from foods that come from animals, such as meats, poultry, fish, egg yolks, and whole-milk products. About 20 percent of our blood cholesterol comes from the cholesterol in the foods you eat. The amount of fat and cholesterol you eat can influence all your blood fats, including blood cholesterol levels.

The problem occurs when there's too much cholesterol circulating in the bloodstream. As you now know, excess cholesterol can lead to atherosclerosis, the plaque-building process that narrows arteries throughout the body and can lead to chest pain, heart attack, or stroke.

# Types of Cholesterol

Just as oil and water do not mix, the same is true for cholesterol and blood. Cholesterol cannot dissolve in blood. To enable cholesterol to travel through the blood, the body coats cholesterol with proteins called *apoproteins*. Once combined with these proteins, another complex protein called a *lipoprotein* is formed. These protein carriers carry cholesterol and *triglycerides* (another type of blood fat) through the bloodstream. There are several different types of lipoproteins. Each affects CHD and heart attack risk differently.

## Low-Density Lipoprotein Cholesterol

This type of lipoprotein is called "bad" cholesterol because it is the main source of cholesterol in the blood and one of the major culprits in the buildup of atherosclerotic plaque. (Remember that LDL is the "bad" cholesterol by associating the "L" with "lousy.") LDL cholesterol carries some 60 to 70 percent of the body's circulating cholesterol.

As LDL cholesterol circulates through the bloodstream, the body uses some of it to build cells. Some of the cholesterol returns to the liver. However, when there is too much LDL cholesterol circulating in the blood, it can slowly build up on the walls of the coronary arteries. The more LDL cholesterol you have in your blood, the higher your risk for CHD and heart attack.

## High-Density Lipoprotein Cholesterol

This is the so-called "good" cholesterol (remember that HDL is the "good" cholesterol by associating the H with "healthy"). High-density lipoprotein particles, which contain mostly protein, carry anywhere from 20 to 30 percent of the cholesterol in the blood. HDL cholesterol is considered "good" because it acts like a trash collector, picking up excess cholesterol from the artery walls and sending it to the liver for disposal. As a result, HDL cholesterol slows plaque growth and may reverse the plaque-building process. Generally, the higher your level

23

## Cholesterol Guidelines

| HDL Cholesterol Levels | |
|---|---|
| High | 60 (higher is better) |
| Low | less than 40 |

| LDL Cholesterol Levels | |
|---|---|
| Ideal | less than 70 |
| Normal | 70–100 |
| Borderline High | 101–130 |
| High | 131–160 |
| Very High | greater than 160 |

| Triglyceride Levels | |
|---|---|
| Normal | less than 150 |
| Borderline High | 150–199 |
| High | 200–499 |
| Very High | greater than 500 |

*Note:* Measurements are expressed in milligrams per deciliter of blood.

of HDL, the lower your risk of heart disease and heart attack. On the other hand, low levels of HDL increase your risk for CHD and heart attack.

### Triglycerides

Triglycerides are another type of blood fat. Most of the body's fat is stored as triglycerides in fat tissue. A small portion of triglycerides circulate in the blood. Triglyceride levels in the blood are related to your consumption of dietary fat and carbohydrates; the amount of alcohol you consume is also a factor. Triglyceride levels are also influenced by genetics.

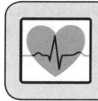

**Heart Notes**

More than half of all Americans have total cholesterol levels higher than 200 mg/dL, putting them at risk for CHD and heart attack.

Heart experts believe that excessive levels of triglycerides may contribute to the fatty deposits that obstruct blood flow and increase the risk for heart attack. A twenty-year study published in the journal *Circulation* found that people with elevated triglycerides have a greater risk of dying from a heart attack, even if their blood cholesterol is normal.

## Cholesterol Creates Plaque Buildup

As excess cholesterol travels in the blood, it is taken up by special cells in the artery walls. This process creates "lumps" in the artery walls that are covered over or encapsulated by fibrous scar tissue. Some of these lumps, called *stable plaques,* become quite large and dramatically narrow or even totally block arteries. When these large blockages reduce the amount of blood getting to the heart, they can cause chest pain, or angina.

*Unstable plaques* are those that are loaded with cholesterol and tend to rupture easily. When unstable plaques burst into the artery channel, they release their cholesterol into the bloodstream. The body responds by triggering a blood clot inside the artery to repair the damage to the inner artery wall. This blood clot may totally block the artery, stopping blood flow and causing a heart attack.

The area of the heart that doesn't receive blood starts to die within twenty minutes, permanently damaging the heart muscle. Even if the clot doesn't cause a heart attack, it can cause disturbances that interfere with the heart's rhythm. This condition can lead to cardiac arrest and death.

Reducing the amount of cholesterol in the blood can help lower the amount of cholesterol in plaques, making them more stable and less likely to burst and trigger a heart attack. Even in people who have already had a heart attack, lowering cholesterol can lower the chance of having another heart attack in the future.

## Factors That Contribute to High Cholesterol

In most cases, there is no single cause of high blood cholesterol. Your blood cholesterol level may be affected by your diet, but it may also be affected by how quickly your body makes LDL cholesterol and how rapidly it gets rid of it.

Following are factors that can contribute to high cholesterol:

### Genetics

Genes you inherit from your family can influence how rapidly your body makes LDL cholesterol and how efficiently it's removed. Your liver can influence your cholesterol levels. Some people—approximately one in 500— have *familial hypercholesterolemia,* an inherited disorder that causes cholesterol levels to be extremely high (350 to 500 mg/dL).

### Diet

What you eat affects your blood cholesterol levels. Saturated fats, especially, will raise your bad cholesterol levels. These fats are found mostly in meats, egg yolks, and dairy products.

### Excess Weight

Excess weight tends to increase LDL cholesterol levels. When your extra pounds are around your waist, your risk for heart disease is even greater. Losing weight can lower "bad" LDL cholesterol levels, raise "good" HDL cholesterol, and reduce triglyceride levels.

## Physical Inactivity

Inactivity can negatively influence your blood cholesterol levels. Regular physical activity can decrease "bad" LDL cholesterol and raise "good" HDL cholesterol levels. For overall cardiovascular health, the American Heart Association (AHA) recommends thirty minutes of moderate exercise five days weekly or twenty-five minutes of vigorous exercise three days weekly. For additional benefit, the AHA recommends moderate to high-intensity muscle training two days per week. To reduce cholesterol or blood pressure, they recommend forty minutes of moderate to vigorous exercise three to four days a week.

## Age

As people get older, their blood cholesterol levels tend to rise. This rise usually levels off at about sixty to sixty-five years of age.

## Menopause

Women's total blood cholesterol levels tend to be lower than those for men of the same age. However, after menopause, women's LDL ("bad") cholesterol increases and their HDL ("good") cholesterol tends to decrease. Some authorities believe this change in cholesterol levels may be one reason why women's risk of heart disease rises sharply after menopause.

## Smoking

Smoking damages the lining of your arteries, leading to a buildup of fatty material which narrows the arteries. This can cause angina, heart attack, or stroke. Smoking can also lower "good" HDL cholesterol levels by as much as 15 percent.

## Stress

It is known that when we are under stress or become angry, the adrenal glands produce excess amounts of the hormones adrenaline and cortisol. These hormones normally circulate in the body, but increased levels are thought to affect cholesterol levels and how the blood clots; it can also increase upper-body fat factors that influence the development of heart disease.

# 4 SYMPTOMS OF CORONARY HEART DISEASE

You could have coronary heart disease and not even know it. Especially in the early stages, you may have no symptoms at all. You may feel fine, unaware that there's a silent time bomb ticking away inside your coronary arteries. As the arteries become narrower and the heart begins to have less and less blood and oxygen available to it, you may experience shortness of breath, periodic pain, tightness, or pressure in the chest. Some people may develop no symptoms. Unfortunately, their first indication that they have CHD is a heart attack.

## Chest Pain

Pressure, pain, or tightness in the chest are the symptoms most commonly associated with CHD. Known as *angina* or *angina pectoris,* this pain occurs when the heart doesn't receive enough blood and oxygen. It is often a recurring pain or discomfort in the chest that occurs when part of the heart doesn't get enough blood. People often describe angina as pressure, squeezing, burning, tightness, or heaviness. Most commonly, the discomfort is felt under the breastbone. However, sometimes people feel discomfort in the shoulders, arms, neck, jaw, or back. Some people also experience numbness in the shoulders, arms, or wrists.

Angina usually lasts no more than five to fifteen minutes. Events that may trigger angina include: exertion or physical stress, eating a heavy meal, exposure to extreme

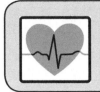

**Heart Notes**

Take angina seriously, especially if you smoke, are overweight, have a family history of heart disease, have high cholesterol, or are a diabetic.

heat or cold, drinking alcohol, and smoking. Angina may be relieved within a few minutes by stopping the stressful activity.

Angina is not a heart attack. Angina attacks usually do not permanently damage the heart muscle. In contrast, during a heart attack, blood flow to part of the heart is partially or completely blocked and the damage to the heart muscle may be serious and is permanent. The pain during a heart attack is usually more severe and lasts longer than angina.

### Other Causes of Chest Pain

Chest pain may also be caused by other serious heart and circulatory problems such as: pericarditis, dissection of the aorta, or pulmonary embolism.

*Pericarditis* is an inflammation of the *pericardium,* the fibrous outer sac that surrounds the heart. The chest pain it causes is usually sharp, even knifelike. It's made worse by taking a deep breath or lying down and it improves when you lean forward.

*Dissection of the aorta* is a tearing of the inner lining of the aorta, the major artery that leads away from the heart. It typically causes back pain, often described as a tearing sensation. This is a life-threatening condition that often requires emergency surgery.

A *pulmonary embolism* is a blood clot in the lung. The pain is located in the chest and typically gets worse when you take a deep breath, or it may cause a feeling of heaviness in the chest—similar to angina. Both angina and pulmonary embolism may cause some degree of breathlessness.

## Types of Angina

Angina is classified as *stable, unstable,* or *variant.*

### Stable angina

If you have stable angina:

- You probably experience chest discomfort when you overexert.

- The pain is relatively predictable and, almost any time you overexert, the pain returns. For instance, you may feel chest pain and tightness when you perform heavy labor such as shoveling snow or during times of emotional stress. Over time, you probably learn to identify what brings on your angina attacks.

### Unstable Angina

Unstable angina is less predictable and is more dangerous because it carries a higher risk of heart attack. Symptoms include:

- new chest pain or discomfort that may come on suddenly during activities that never caused problems before

- a changing pattern of stable angina (pain occurring at lower levels of activity, more often, or more severely)

- chest pain that occurs at rest or that wakes one from sleep

Although both stable and unstable anginas are caused by the atherosclerotic plaques of CHD, the plaque in unstable angina is more often related to rupturing on the inner surface of the artery. When this happens, the body forms a blood clot to repair the damage. If the clot is large enough, it may block blood flow and cause a heart attack. Unstable angina can also cause severe heart rhythm problems or sudden cardiac death, in which the heart muscle simply stops functioning.

*Variant Angina*

A less common type of angina is called *variant angina*. In this form of angina, the muscle fibers surrounding the coronary arteries go into spasm, which causes a blood vessel to become very narrow or even close off completely. About 65 percent of people who suffer variant angina have severe coronary atherosclerotic plaque in at least one major coronary vessel. The spasm usually occurs very close to the artery blockage.

Variant angina attacks often occur without exertion or other apparent cause, or they may be brought on by stress, exposure to cold, or smoking. Variant angina attacks are usually severe and last only a short time. They often occur at rest, between midnight and 8:00 A.M.; these attacks usually wake a person from sleep with the discomfort. During attacks, abnormal heart rhythms can cause one to lose consciousness.

## Angina Is a Warning

Regardless of the type of angina you may have, it has the same cause: the heart's demand for oxygen is not being met due to atherosclerotic plaque. Angina is a warning from your heart. Angina may not indicate that you are about to have a heart attack, but it does mean that you may have underlying CHD and that you may be at increased risk for heart attack.

If you experience angina, don't ignore it. Angina is your body's cry for help. See your doctor immediately for evaluation. Don't wait a few days or a few weeks for an appointment to address the symptoms. After your condition is properly diagnosed, your doctor can prescribe lifestyle changes and medications. Medical procedures may also be recommended; these include the placement of a stent or possibly bypass surgery. Both of these procedures treat clogged arteries and can relieve your discomfort.

### Learn the Pattern of Your Angina

After your doctor has evaluated and treated your condition, try to learn what brings on and what relieves attacks. Pay attention to what your angina attacks feel like, how long episodes usually last, and how medication affects them. Watch for changes in the pattern of angina. See your doctor right away if your angina:

- becomes more frequent
- lasts longer
- occurs at rest

Know the symptoms of a heart attack (*see* chapter 5). Call 911 for emergency medical help immediately if the pattern of your angina changes sharply or if you have any symptoms of a heart attack.

### Not All Chest Pain Is Angina

Your pain is probably not angina if:

- it lasts for less than thirty seconds
- taking a deep breath relieves it
- it goes away after drinking a glass of water
- it disappears if you change body positions
- it's localized on the surface of your chest and you can reproduce it by touching a particular spot

If you have any doubt, see your doctor.

## Silent Ischemia

When there is a temporary shortage of blood and oxygen to the heart without any symptoms, it's called *silent ischemia.* It can occur when a coronary artery is narrowed by atherosclerotic plaque, or spasm, or when the heart's oxygen demand exceeds the supply. The problem with silent ischemia is that it is silent; there is no pain, no discomfort, no warning until there's a heart attack.

# 5 UNDERSTANDING HEART ATTACK

Every forty seconds, someone in the United States suffers a heart attack, also known as *myocardial infarction* or *MI*. Just under 800,000 people in the United States have heart attacks annually. The average age of a first heart attack among men is sixty-six. For women, the average age is seventy. The most common cause of heart attacks is coronary heart disease, which is influenced by lifestyle choices.

Fortunately, heart attacks are not usually fatal, and knowing the signs and symptoms of a heart attack can help save your life or the life of a loved one. The key is getting medical attention immediately.

**What Happens During a Heart Attack?**
A heart attack occurs when the blood supply to part of the heart is severely reduced or completely blocked. This occurs when one of the coronary arteries supplying the heart becomes severely narrowed or blocked, usually from a combination of too much atherosclerotic plaque and a blood clot. Typically, when plaque tears or ruptures, the cholesterol core of the plaque is exposed to circulating blood cells *(platelets)*. In response, the body forms a blood clot. If this blood clot severely restricts or blocks the blood supply to part of the heart, a heart attack can occur.

If heart cells are denied blood and oxygen for a prolonged period of time, they suffer irreversible injury

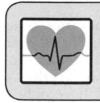

### Heart Notes

Sixty percent of people who die of a heart attack die within the first hour. Get help fast! Time is critical with a heart attack.

and begin to die. Depending on how much of the heart is damaged, a heart attack can cause the heart to be unable to pump enough blood to the body (heart failure) or cause death.

Heart attacks can also occur when a coronary artery temporarily goes into spasm. This can reduce or even stop blood flow to part of the heart, especially if the coronary artery is already narrowed by atherosclerotic plaque. Many factors contribute to spasm, including the local release of chemical substances that may trigger spasm and the ability of the artery to contract. Both normal and diseased arteries may develop spasm. If the spasm is severe enough, a heart attack can result.

## Heart Attack Symptoms

Common symptoms of a heart attack are:

- uncomfortable pressure, tightness, fullness, squeezing, or pain in the center of the chest
- pain that lasts more than a few minutes (thirty minutes to several hours) or goes away and comes back
- pain that spreads to the shoulders, neck, or arms
- light-headedness or fainting
- nausea
- profuse sweating
- shortness of breath

## Less Typical Symptoms of a Heart Attack

Not everyone experiences a heart attack the same way. Even if you've had one or more heart attacks, another attack may feel different. Some people feel the classic, heavy, heart attack chest pain. People often describe it as a "vice squeezing my chest." Others may have only a vague sense of discomfort, indigestion, breathlessness, or dizziness. People who have diabetes, women, and people over the age of seventy-five often have symptoms that are less typical, such as:

- vague chest pain
- stomach or abdominal pain
- nausea or dizziness, without chest pain
- shortness of breath or difficulty breathing, without chest pain
- anxiety without obvious cause
- impending sense of doom
- weakness or fatigue
- erratic heartbeat
- cold sweating
- paleness
- frequent angina not caused by exertion
- dry mouth or cough, usually with shortness of breath

## Immediate Medical Care Is Critical

When a person has a heart attack, time is critical. The longer an artery is blocked, the more damage to the heart muscle and the greater the risk of permanent disability or even death. Additionally, the heart's rhythm and pumping may become scrambled. Instead of pumping in a synchronized fashion, the heart may twitch erratically *(ventricular fibrillation)* and becomes unable to pump blood. If ventricular fibrillation lasts longer than a few minutes, it can cause death.

## Heart Attack Warning Signs

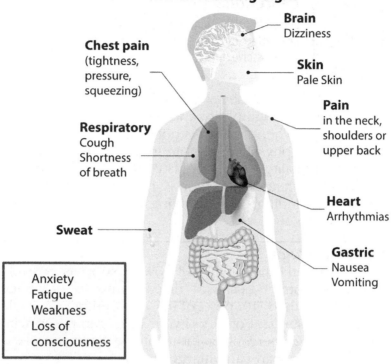

**Brain**
Dizziness

**Chest pain**
(tightness,
pressure,
squeezing)

**Skin**
Pale Skin

**Pain**
in the neck,
shoulders or
upper back

**Respiratory**
Cough
Shortness
of breath

**Heart**
Arrhythmias

**Sweat**

**Gastric**
Nausea
Vomiting

Anxiety
Fatigue
Weakness
Loss of
consciousness

### Don't Wait to Get Help

Many people mistake the symptoms of a heart attack for indigestion or stress and they delay getting to a hospital. This is a dangerous and often fatal mistake. Anyone with heart attack symptoms should be rushed to the nearest hospital by ambulance—do not have a friend or relative drive you. Call 911. An ambulance arrives with paramedics who can begin life-saving care immediately upon arrival.

### Get to an Emergency Room

If you get to an emergency room fast, doctors can use a variety of techniques and medications to help restore blood flow to the part of the heart that is damaged during

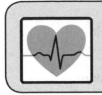

**Heart Notes**

Remember this important tip: Chewing aspirin during a heart attack can save your life. Aspirin thins the blood and helps dissolve clots.

the heart attack. Whenever possible, standard treatment involves balloon angioplasty and the insertion of stents.

However, when stenting is not available at your treatment center, a physician may arrange for an emergency transfer to a facility for angioplasty and possibly surgery. If travel to a treatment center is not feasible, alternate treatments including clot-dissolving medications may be considered.

### Saving Heart Muscle

Restoring the heart's blood flow as soon as possible is vitally important because "time is muscle." Damage to even less than 10 percent of the ventricle muscle decreases the amount of blood your heart can pump with each beat. If 25 percent or more of the heart muscle is damaged, your heart can enlarge and be unable to pump adequately. When 40 percent or more of the heart muscle is damaged, shock or death may result. The sooner the doctors can restore blood flow to your heart, the more likely you'll survive.

Nowadays, an interventional cardiologist's goal is to open a blocked artery within ninety minutes (preferably sixty) from the first medical contact in an emergency room. Results are best when an experienced team performs the procedure to open the blocked artery and insert a stent (propping open the arteries with fine wire mesh). Opening the artery within ninety minutes after arriving at an emergency room (preferably from the time of first medical contact) improves your chances of surviving a heart attack. We'll talk more about procedures to place stents in chapter 9.

## Surviving a Heart Attack

Knowing what to do in the case of a heart attack can mean the difference between life and death. The following guidelines can help save the life of someone having a heart attack.

- Keep a list of emergency rescue numbers handy. Call 911 or other emergency medical numbers immediately if you experience symptoms.

- Know which medical centers offer twenty-four-hour cardiac care and which one is closest to your home and office.

- Know and recognize the symptoms of heart attack. About half of all heart attack victims have warning signs hours, days, or even weeks before an attack. Be aware that not all heart attacks involve the classic crushing chest pain.

- Chew one regular-strength aspirin (unless you are allergic) if you experience heart attack symptoms. It will help break up clots if you're having an attack. When taken during an attack, aspirin can decrease death rates by about 25 percent. Chewing the aspirin speeds its absorption. Do not take aspirin if you have a history of bleeding or are allergic to it.

- If your doctor has given you nitroglycerine tablets, place one under your tongue when symptoms begin. Repeat every five minutes for a total of three doses. Do not take nitroglycerine if your doctor hasn't prescribed it for you or if you feel dizzy, unless you're directed to do so by a health care professional. Taking nitroglycerine for some types of heart conditions can be dangerous. Do not take nitroglycerine if you have taken erectile dysfunction medications Viagra, Cialis, or Levitra within twenty-four to forty-eight hours.

## Sudden Cardiac Death

*Sudden cardiac death (SCD)* is the most common reason people die from CHD. Sudden cardiac death is the abrupt, total loss of heart function in someone with or without diagnosed heart disease. Such death is usually unexpected. About half of all deaths from atherosclerosis occur suddenly.

People who die from sudden cardiac death almost always have underlying heart disease. Most often, it is atherosclerosis. In about 90 percent of those who die suddenly, two or more major coronary arteries are narrowed by atherosclerotic plaque; however, one blocked vessel can also cause death. Two-thirds of SCD victims have heart damage from previous heart attacks. The first six months following a heart attack is a high-risk time for people to die from SCD.

Sudden cardiac death has the same risk factors as coronary heart disease. Strategies to reduce risk factors for CHD and reduce or prevent atherosclerosis can help reduce the risk of sudden death.

## Recovering from a Heart Attack

If you have had a heart attack, you may be able to return to an active life and return to work in two weeks to three months depending on the severity of your heart attack and type of job you have. Lifestyle changes are recommended, including a heart-healthy diet and a moni-tored exercise program. Frequently, you'll be prescribed new medications such as aspirin and other blood-thin-ning medications, beta-blockers (for heart protection and blood pressure), statins (for high cholesterol), and ACE inhibitors or ARBs (angiotensin receptor blockers—for heart healing and blood pressure).

Also, don't neglect your emotional state. Talk with your doctor about the emotions you are feeling. He or she may prescribe an antidepressant.

# 6 HEART DISEASE IN WOMEN

**M**any people believe that coronary heart disease affects mostly men; however, heart disease (especially CHD) and stroke are the leading causes of death for women in the United States. Every year, heart disease and stroke kill more than half a million women in the United States, nearly twice as many as from all forms of cancer.

The risk is even greater for minority women. The rate of death from heart disease for black women is 69 percent higher than for white women. Black women are more likely to die of a heart attack before menopause, too.

Women over sixty-five are most vulnerable to CHD; however, middle-aged women between forty-five and sixty-four are at risk, as well. One in nine American women in this age group show signs of CHD.

## Under-Diagnosed: Heart Attacks in Women

Unfortunately, a woman may be unaware that she has a buildup of artery-clogging plaque and may first learn she has heart disease when she has a potentially fatal heart attack. Two-thirds of women who die of a heart attack have no prior symptoms, compared to only half of men who die from a heart attack.

Women are also less likely than men to get the right diagnosis and treatment for CHD. The American Heart Association concluded that both women and their doctors often attribute women's chest pains to non-heart causes.

**Heart Attack Symptoms in Women**

Women often do not realize they're having a heart attack. These symptoms can be more subtle.

- Chronic breathlessness or difficulty breathing
- Unexplained dizziness or blackouts
- Swelling in the ankles or lower legs
- Rapid heartbeat
- Nausea or upset stomach

This can result in dangerous misdiagnoses. Part of this may be due to the fact that women are more apt to have subtle, atypical heart attack symptoms. While some women have the classic heart attack chest pain that radiates to the shoulders, neck, or arms, many have less typical chest discomfort or abdominal pain, difficulty breathing, and other less recognizable symptoms.

A type of heart attack, a *spontaneous coronary dissection (SCAD)*, occurs when there is a sudden tear with the layers of one or more arteries to the heart. This may occur in women who often have none of the traditional risk factors for CHD. The possible symptoms include: chest discomfort, indigestion, shortness of breath. Always remember that these symptoms may be a heart attack and should never be ignored.

Unfortunately, most women are not aware of their risk for heart disease. A poll conducted for the American Heart Association found that most women do not recognize that heart disease is women's leading health problem. In fact, fewer than one in ten women believe heart disease is their greatest health threat.

## Heart Attack Symptoms in Women

Sometimes, women do not realize they're having a heart attack because their symptoms can be subtler than the classic symptoms. Women's symptoms may include:

- chronic breathlessness or difficulty breathing
- unexplained dizziness or blackouts
- swelling in the ankles or lower legs
- rapid heartbeat
- nausea or upset stomach

## Risk Factors for CHD in Women

Because of the physical differences in men and women, it shouldn't surprise us that CHD develops a bit differently in women and men. Some of the risk factors for CHD impact women differently from men.

### Smoking

Women who smoke twenty cigarettes or more per day are six times more likely to have a heart attack than women who never smoked. For men, the risk was 2.8 times greater when compared to nonsmoking males.

### Increasing Age

Compared with men, women's risk of heart disease is relatively low until menopause. The female hormone estrogen may have a protective effect by raising a woman's "good" HDL cholesterol and lowering "bad" LDL cholesterol. However, after menopause and the subsequent decrease in estrogen, a woman's risk of heart attack rises. At age sixty-five, a woman's risk for heart attack is nearly that of men.

### High Cholesterol/Triglycerides

Total cholesterol levels are not as strong an indicator of heart disease for women as for men. For women, it appears that HDL ("good") levels are more important. Low levels of HDL in women appear to be a greater risk for CHD and heart attack for women older than sixty-five than in men of the same age. Some heart disease experts suggest that the national guideline of HDL levels of less

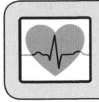 Heart disease kills more women than all cancers combined. Sixty-four percent of women who die suddenly of coronary heart disease had no previous symptoms.

than 35 mg/dL as an independent risk factor for CHD may be too low for women. They suggest 45 mg/dL or even higher HDL is a better standard.

### Diabetes

As mentioned previously, diabetes is a major risk factor for CHD and heart attack for both men and women, but it impacts women's risk even more dramatically. Having diabetes increases a woman's CHD risk by three to seven times compared with a twofold to threefold increase in men. This may be because diabetes in women has an especially negative effect on blood fats and blood pressure.

### Hormone Replacement Therapy

For many years, doctors believed that *hormone replacement therapy (HRT)* provided postmenopausal women with protection against heart disease and heart attacks. However, research from the large-scale Heart and Estrogen Replacement Study (HERS) found that HRT provides no protective benefit against heart disease in women. Another study, the Estrogen Replacement and Atherosclerosis (ERA) Trial, found HRT did not slow the progression of atherosclerosis in women with heart disease or blood vessel disease.

The American Heart Association advises doctors against prescribing HRT for the sole purpose of preventing heart attacks and strokes in women with heart disease. Instead, they recommend women with heart disease reduce their risk of heart attack and stroke by making lifestyles changes such as quitting smoking, losing weight,

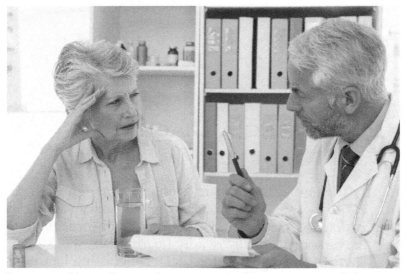

Symptoms of heart disease often go unnoticed amoung women. Talk to your doctor about any possible symptoms, especially if you have a family history of heart disease.

and exercising regularly. These are considered first-line CHD therapies.

Medications to reduce high cholesterol and/or high blood pressure can also help lower risk. There is evidence that statin medications, which lower cholesterol, are under-prescribed in women and could help lower cholesterol levels better than hormone replacement therapy. Talk to your doctor about whether HRT is right for you to treat other issues such as symptoms of menopause.

## Get Help Immediately

As stressed throughout this book, call 911, and seek emergency medical care any time you suspect a heart attack. The sooner medical care is received, the greater are your chances for avoiding damage to heart muscle.

## 7 GETTING A DIAGNOSIS

A number of tests are available to diagnose heart disease. The sooner your coronary heart disease is diagnosed, the sooner you can begin treatment to help prevent a potentially deadly heart attack.

There is no single test for CHD. Diagnosing heart disease can be a complex task because more than one type of heart disease may be present. Additionally, you may have other health problems that make it more difficult to make a precise diagnosis. Your diagnosis will be based on your medical history, a physical examination, and diagnostic tests.

### Your Medical History

The first thing your doctor will likely do is review your medical history and conduct a medical interview. Your medical history will include a number of questions about illnesses, and surgeries that you or close family members have had.

Providing complete and thorough information will help your doctor get a more accurate picture of your health. During the interview, your doctor will review your medical history with you and ask you a number of questions about your current state of health, including any symptoms you may be having. You should be prepared to answer questions such as:

- Have you or anyone in your family had a heart attack, stroke, or circulatory problem?

46

- What medications do you take?
- Have you ever had an abnormal electrocardiogram or exercise stress test?
- Have you ever taken heart medications or cholesterol-lowering medications?
- Describe your symptoms. When do these symptoms occur?
- What makes these symptoms better or worse?

## Physical Examination

After your doctor has thoroughly interviewed you about your medical history and your symptoms, he or she will conduct a physical exam. This includes checking your vital signs—pulse, blood pressure, breathing or respiratory rate.

If you have no CHD symptoms, your doctor will check for signs of poor circulation at various points in your body. Using a stethoscope, he or she will listen to your heart for irregular sounds and will examine your neck, abdomen, and elsewhere for evidence of what are called *bruits,* which are noises produced by turbulent blood flow through narrowed arteries. Your doctor will also listen to your lungs, looking for signs of extra fluid buildup. By carefully observing the veins in your neck while you're in various positions, the doctor can detect elevated pressures on the right side of the heart.

He or she will also look for skin that is cool and pale or bluish *(cyanotic),* a sign of poor circulation. Because severe atherosclerosis in the legs can cause hair loss and thickening of the toenails, the doctor will examine your feet and legs. He or she will also look for evidence of swelling *(edema),* especially in your feet, ankles, and legs.

## Diagnostic Tests for CHD

The diagnostic tests your doctor uses will depend on your symptoms, your medical history, your risk factors,

---

**Common Diagnostic Tests for CHD**

- Blood tests (lipid profile, blood count, chemistries)
- Electrocardiography (ECG)
- Chest X-ray
- Nuclear scanning (SPECT and MUGA) and stress testing
- Catheterization and angiography
- Advance imaging (CT, PET, MRI)

---

and the results of your physical exam. The diagnostic tests selected will be tailored for you. Regardless of whether or not you have CHD symptoms, you'll probably need more than one diagnostic test. Fortunately, many of the tests for CHD are noninvasive—they're done outside the body and are painless.

### Chest X-ray

Your doctor may order a chest X-ray to look at the size and shape of your heart and major blood vessels. A chest X-ray also lets the doctor examine your lungs. If your heart isn't pumping strongly enough, for instance, fluid may leak into the air sacs of the lungs. (This is called *pulmonary edema*).

For this test, you'll be asked to remove your clothing and jewelry from the waist up and put on a hospital gown. You'll stand against a plate that holds the X-ray film and hold your arms out to the sides. You'll be asked to take a breath and hold it, which helps the heart and lungs appear clearly on the X-ray.

Having a chest X-ray with today's low-dose machines is quite safe. However, if you're pregnant, or think you might be, be sure to tell your doctor before having a chest X-ray. Risk to an unborn baby is low, but special precautions should be taken to protect the baby from exposure. A chest X-ray during pregnancy is done only when absolutely necessary.

## Electrocardiogram

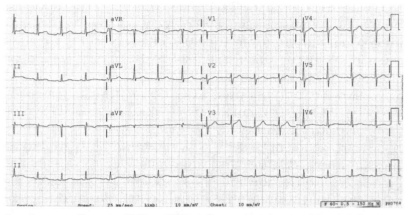

An electrocardiogram (ECG or EKG) reflects the overall health of the heart muscle and whether it's beating normally. The test does not tell whether arteries are blocked.

*Electrocardiogram*

One of the most common tests for heart disease, an *electrocardiogram (ECG,* also called *EKG)* records the electrical activity of the heart. Your doctor will likely order an ECG if you have CHD symptoms such as chest pain, shortness of breath, palpitations (rapid fluttering of the heart), or fainting. Some doctors like to do an ECG on anyone over age forty during routine examinations.

The ECG is painless and takes less than ten minutes. You lie on an examination table while a nurse or technician attaches twelve small discs (electrodes) at various points on your body. These electrodes are attached to wires, which are attached to the electrocardiogram machine; as you lie quietly, these electrodes pick up the electrical impulses of your heart. As the machine records your heart's activity, the results are recorded as "waves" displayed on a monitor or printed on paper.

The ECG provides valuable information about your heart's rate and rhythm, and whether you've previously had a heart attack or have structural abnormalities. How-

49

ever, like most tests, it's not without limitations. A normal ECG doesn't rule out CHD. In fact, you may have a totally normal ECG but still have a 90 percent narrowing of a major coronary artery. Unfortunately, changes in ECG results often don't occur until atherosclerosis is very severe or after structural damage has occurred.

Likewise, an abnormal ECG doesn't mean you definitely have CHD, particularly if you don't have CHD symptoms or risk factors. ECG abnormalities can be caused by non-heart problems such as long-standing high blood pressure, lung disease, and abnormal electrolytes in the blood. *Electrolytes* are minerals (sodium, potassium, calcium, and magnesium) that stimulate muscles and nerves. They also regulate fluids throughout your body, which affect cellular function, blood volume, and blood pressure.

### Echocardiogram

An *echocardiogram* is a noninvasive procedure that uses high-pitched ultrasound waves to show a picture of the heart. (This is the same ultrasound technology that is used to view a baby inside a mother's uterus.) An echocardiogram provides precise information about your heart's function, its valves, and adjacent structures. During an echocardiogram, sound waves produce an image of the beating heart. The test measures heart function and can detect narrowing arteries when combined with stress testing.

As the ultrasound detects heart sounds, it displays an image of the blood flowing between different chambers of the heart. A color map and other precise measurements assess the severity of any narrowing or leakage in one or more heart valves. It can also measure the pressure inside the lungs.

Your echocardiogram is usually done in a cardiologist's office, in a laboratory, or in a hospital. You don't need to follow any special instructions before having this test.

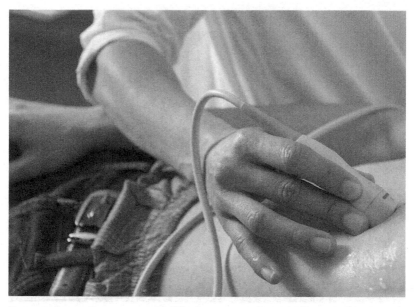

For an echocardiogram, a wandlike instrument is moved across the chest. It uses high-frequency sound waves (ultrasound) to produce a picture of the heart at work. The test shows the size, structure, and movement of various parts of the heart.

For this test, you'll be asked to remove your clothing from the waist up and put on a hospital gown or drape. You'll lie down on your back or left side. A technician will apply a special gel to your chest; the gel improves the transmission of ultrasound waves. Then, a doctor, nurse, or lab technician will move a handheld instrument (a *transducer*) over your chest. The transducer is attached to a monitoring screen. The examination is painless and will take fifteen to sixty minutes. There is no known risk to having an ultrasound.

Certain conditions make it difficult to get a clear ultrasound image. Such conditions include:

- having lung disease (such as emphysema)
- being very overweight
- having spinal or chest wall abnormalities

51

**Results of Echocardiogram**

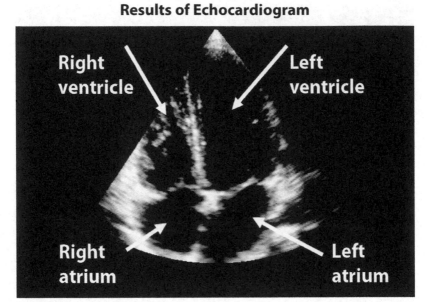

During an echocardiogram, sound waves produce an image of the beating heart. The test measures heart function and can detect narrowing arteries when combined with stress testing.

- having very large breasts or breast implants
- having had chest or heart surgery or a chest injury
- being on a ventilator

Sometimes doctors use *echocardiography* to view the heart under stress. This test includes a number of steps. First, your doctor will perform a resting echocardiogram. Next, you may be asked to walk on a treadmill or ride a stationary bike; an alternative to the treadmill or bike, you may be given a medication, *dobutamine,* injected intravenously; it causes the heart to beat faster and stronger for a few minutes.

Immediately after the exercise is performed another echocardiogram is taken and the ultrasound images are captured as a digital recording. This enables doctors to compare ultrasound images of the heart both at rest and under stress.

If you are scheduled for a stress echocardiogram, you may be asked to refrain from eating or drinking for several hours before the test. It's a good idea to ask your doctor if it's okay to take your routine prescriptions or over-the-counter medications, or herbal supplements, on the day of the test.

A specialized type of echocardiogram, the *trans-esophageal echocardiogram (TEE)*, magnifies the heart's structures (including the valves). This test can detect blood clots that are hiding in the top left chamber of the heart. These hidden clots can travel and may cause a stroke. TEE is also used in people during open-heart surgery to check the valves and heart muscle function.

Unlike other forms of echocardiography, TEE is somewhat invasive. The test takes approximately twenty minutes and is usually done on an outpatient basis. The throat is numbed with a local anesthesia and a tube is passed through the esophagus, which lies directly behind the heart. The tube contains a tiny ultrasound crystal that reflects an ultrasound image.

### Exercise Stress Test

The *exercise stress test* measures how your heart muscle functions under stress, or in this case, exercise. It's also referred to as a *treadmill test*. First, electrodes are attached to your torso to record heart activity. Then, you walk on a treadmill or pedal a stationary bike. Because this test produces higher heart rates than the resting ECG, it's better for detecting problems such as poor circulation and insufficient blood supply to the coronary arteries.

The exercise test can also detect exercise-related heart rhythm disturbances and abnormalities in blood pressure response. If you've had a heart attack or you're already being treated for heart problems with medications, your doctor may order periodic stress ECG tests to check for coronary artery obstructions. If your doctor orders an exercise stress test for you:

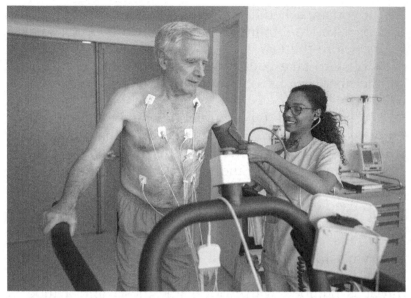

Exercise makes your heart work harder. For an exercise stress test, you walk on a treadmill or ride a stationary bike while blood flow within your heart is monitored by and ECG.

- Eat only a light breakfast or lunch before taking the test. Allow at least two hours between your meal and your exercise stress test.

- Take your medications as usual, unless directed otherwise. Some people need to stop taking their medications a day or two before the test—your doctor will tell you if that's necessary. (Some tests are designed to detect a problem and medications are withheld. Other tests are given to see how well the person is protected by medications.)

- Wear comfortable clothing and walking shoes.

- You'll be asked to walk on a treadmill or pedal a stationary bike for five to fifteen minutes. The rest of the time you'll be monitored at rest.

Let the doctor, nurse, or technician know immediately if you feel chest discomfort or shortness of breath during the test. For most people, undergoing an exercise stress test is safe. Because the test stresses the heart, there is a small risk of suffering a heart attack or serious rhythm disturbance, but the risk is slight. Your doctor, nurses, and the technicians on hand are trained to handle any type of heart emergency that might occur.

The exercise stress test is not perfect—it gives only an indication of whether you have blockages in any of the three major coronary vessels. An artery must be at least 50 percent blocked for the test to detect a blockage. This test detects blockages in about 67 percent of those who have blockages in one of the three major arteries.

When the test is negative, it does not give any information about the presence or absence of plaque buildup in arteries. Your doctor will interpret the results of your exercise test together with your symptoms, your medical history, your risk factors, and other test results.

### Ambulatory ECG

A variation on the exercise stress test is the *ambulatory ECG* (also called *Holter monitoring,* named for its inventor). It monitors the heart continuously during a twenty-four- to forty-eight-hour period. You'll keep the device on even when you're sleeping. This test can help detect heart problems that seem to come and go. If you undergo this test, several electrodes will be attached to your chest so that a small portable digital recording device can record your heart's activity.

An ambulatory ECG can detect abnormal heart rhythms and changes related to lack of blood flow. The doctor will also likely ask you to keep an activity diary, which can be compared with the test results to determine whether the symptoms correspond with the ECG abnormalities.

## Nuclear Stress Test Results

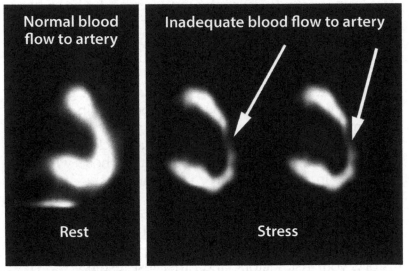

Normal blood flow to artery

Inadequate blood flow to artery

Rest

Stress

On the left, a nuclear stress test shows normal blood flow at rest. The photo on the right shows where there is a lack of blood flow during exercise.

### Nuclear Stress Test

Several types of nuclear scans are available to help doctors determine whether the heart is receiving enough blood flow under stress. Additionally, a doctor may order nuclear scans to monitor the effectiveness of medication or to measure improvement in blood flow to the heart following treatment such as angioplasty or bypass surgery.

The *nuclear stress test* measures blood flow while you are at rest and while you are exerting yourself. This test has a greater chance of detecting blockages compared to an exercise stress test. A nuclear stress test uses radioactive dye and a special camera to take pictures that show the blood flow to your heart.

The nuclear stress test is almost the same as the exercise stress test. However, just before the end of the exercise part of the test, your physician will give you an injection of a radioactive substance. Then, you'll be asked to lie on a table and a special camera will take pictures of your heart; the test will send pictures of your heart to a television monitor for the doctor to view.

A blockage must be fairly severe—at least 50 percent blocked—before it can be detected with nuclear scanning. Scans can detect narrowing in approximately 85–90 percent of people with serious blockages. A negative test can rule out severe blockages in most people, but it doesn't totally eliminate the possibility of a severe blockage (plaque) in the arteries.

If you're pregnant or think you may be, you should avoid nuclear tests.

### Single Proton Emission Computed Tomography (SPECT)

The *single photon emission computed tomography (SPECT)* is one of the most widely used nuclear scan tests. It shows how well blood flows to the heart muscle and how well regions of the heart muscle are functioning. For this test, you'll be given an injection of a radioactive tracer, which allows doctors to see the blood flowing into your heart. While you're lying on a table, a machine will pass over your chest area as it takes images. After the images are captured, a sophisticated computer provides pictures that enable a doctor to see any blood flow problems with the heart at rest and during exercise.

### Pharmacologic Nuclear Stress Test

For individuals who are unable to walk on a treadmill or pedal a stationary bike, the stress test can be done with a scan and a medication that simulates stress on the heart. The test is called a *pharmacologic nuclear stress test*. It may be recommended if you have any of the following conditions:

- chest pain (angina) at rest
- potentially life-threatening heart rhythm problems
- infection, inflammation, or swelling of the heart sac, heart muscle, or heart valves

- a tear on the inner lining of the aorta
- blood clots in the lungs
- other serious or acute illness

## Cardiac Positron-Emission Tomography

A *cardiac positron-emission tomography (PET) scan* is a high-tech nuclear scan that takes computerized pictures of your heart. For a PET scan, you're asked to remove your clothes above the waist and lie on a scanning table, which slides through a large tube-like machine—the PET scanner. Doctors can measure blood flow and metabolism (inner workings of cells) in the heart. This part of the test takes ten to fifteen minutes. Then, you'll be given an injection of a radioactive tracer; after about forty-five minutes, after the tracer has circulated into the bloodstream, more pictures will be taken.

This technology is a very accurate, noninvasive way to detect CHD. It can also identify injured heart tissue. The widespread use of PET has been limited, in part because it's expensive; however its availability has been increasing.

A PET scan is especially useful in people who are overweight and in women in whom breast tissue obscures the view on standard SPECT imaging. Other patients who may be candidates include those who cannot walk on a treadmill due to such ailments as orthopedic problems, chronic lung disease, or peripheral artery disease (PAD).

## Multi-Gated Acquisition

The *multi-gated acquisition (MUGA)* is another nuclear test used to assess heart muscle function at rest and under stress. The test shows doctors whether areas of the heart have been damaged by a previous heart attack or whether the blood flow to the heart is impaired. For a resting stress test, you'll be given an injection of a radioactive solution and you will be asked to lie on a special table; a camera will take images of your heart.

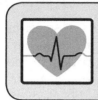 Imaging tests (scans) give doctors an indication of whether you have a serious blockage. The scans are not as helpful if you are at low risk for CHD and have a minor blockage.

If you're taking a stress test, you'll be moved to another table, which has pedals at the end of it. You'll be asked to lie on the table and pedal as if you are riding a bicycle. As you're pedaling, images will be taken of your heart. This test also tells how effectively blood is being pumped from the lower chambers of your heart. The MUGA exercise testing is mostly used to evaluate the heart muscle function.

## Advanced Imaging Diagnostic Tests

Developments in technology have allowed for even more sophisticated imaging of the heart, and, in some cases, may enable doctors to diagnose CHD before a person has symptoms.

### X-ray Computed Tomography

*X-ray computed tomography* (also known as a *CT* or *CAT scan*) produces images of the chest, including the heart, lungs, and major blood vessels. This scan is especially helpful in evaluating diseases of the large blood vessels, masses or tumors in the heart, and diseases of the heart sac or pericardium. It's also helpful in diagnosing blood clots of the lung or tears of the aorta.

The images are produced as an X-ray beam passes through the body. Unlike a regular X-ray machine, the CT X-ray machine rotates rapidly around the body. This allows images to be captured from various angles. A computer then combines the images and produces a detailed cross section of the body. Though there is a small amount of exposure to radiation, all CT scans are painless and involve little risk.

## Coronary Calcium Scoring

*Coronary calcium scoring* (uses 64-slice CT scanner or higher resolution scanners like the 320-slice scanner) is a specialized type of CT scan that can help determine whether you have plaque buildup in your arteries. A cardiologist is looking for plaque, but calcium is the element that shows up in the test; the calcium and the quantity of it is an important indicator of CHD and may predict heart attack risk. In many instances, the test can diagnose atherosclerosis before blockages become severe.

When plaque builds, the blood vessel walls are continually being injured and the body is constantly attempting to heal the injuries. As the body tries to repair the damaged area, calcium is deposited as a result of inflammation. On routine X-rays, this hard calcium shows up only at a very late stage. With coronary calcium scoring, calcium deposits can be detected and measured at an earlier stage. In fact, calcium scoring can determine the presence of CHD even when the arteries are less than 50 percent narrowed, something that many standard cardiac diagnostic tests are unable to do.

This screening study may be recommended if you have risk factors for CHD but no symptoms yet. People who are likely candidates for coronary calcium scoring include:

- men age forty-five and older and women age fifty-five and older
- women who are postmenopausal
- people with a family history of heart disease
- past or present smokers
- people who have a sedentary lifestyle
- people who have a stressful lifestyle
- people with diabetes
- people with high blood pressure

- people with high ("bad") LDL cholesterol or low ("good") HDL cholesterol
- people who are overweight or obese
- people who suffer from other vascular diseases (such as carotid artery narrowing)

*Note:* If you're pregnant or think you might be pregnant, inform your doctor before having this test. It should be postponed until after delivery.

A coronary calcium scoring test doesn't require any special preparation, although you may be asked to avoid caffeine and smoking for four hours prior to the test. If your heartbeat is rapid, you may be given a drug to slow the rate. Performed in the same manner as a standard CT scan, coronary calcium scoring is quick, painless, and involves minimal risk. The results of the test—your calcium score—indicate the amount of calcification in your arteries. The results may be listed as:

- no evidence of plaque
- minimal evidence of plaque
- mild evidence of plaque
- moderate evidence of plaque
- extensive evidence of plaque

Although coronary calcium scoring can be an indication of your risk for CHD, it has limitations. For instance, calcium deposits don't always signify a blockage in the arteries, and not all blockages contain calcium. In addition, the test is unable to detect soft plaque, the earliest form of atherosclerosis. For the coronary scoring test, a 64-slice CT scanner or a 320-slice CT scanner is used.

### 320-Slice Computed Tomography Angiography

This test is a remarkable advance in CT scanning. *The 320-slice computed tomography angiography (CTA) is able to take nearly two hundred images of the heart per second, far faster than standard CT scanners. The speed*

## 320-Slice CTA Scan

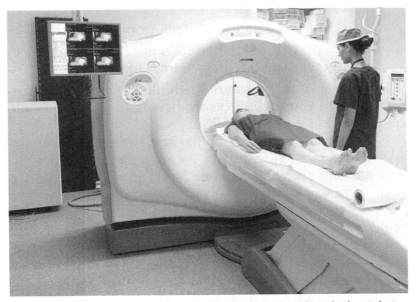

A noninvasive diagnostic test, the 320-slice CTA scan provides a high-resolution image of the heart, helping doctors determine whether any narrowing in the arteries has occurred.

of the 320-Slice CT scanner allows it to virtually "freeze-motion" images of the heart and arteries. Doctors can see, in exact detail, where blood flows within the arteries and determine whether there's a blockage.

When results of a 320-slice CT scan show no blockages in the arteries, it reduces the need for more-invasive diagnostic procedures, such as catheterization and angiography, which are explained later in this chapter. The CTA is a quick, painless procedure that involves placing an IV in the arm to administer a contrast material (X-ray dye) to improve the view of the heart and arteries. You may be given a medication to slow your heartbeat so the motion of your heart is reduced.

After the scan begins, you'll be asked to hold your breath for only a few seconds, as opposed to the twenty-five to forty seconds normally required for standard CT scans. The procedure poses little risk other than a small amount of radiation and the rare side effects associated with the X-ray dye including allergic reaction and kidney injury.

Despite its many benefits, this imaging technique isn't recommended for everyone. Certain situations can reduce the accuracy of the test or can make it difficult to see inside the arteries. Such situations include moderate or heavy calcification in the arteries (a common development if you have CHD), having a stent in an artery, and having a metal heart valve.

### Fractional Flow Reserve Derived from Coronary Computed Angiography

A newer test, called *fractional flow reserve derived from coronary computed angiography (FFR CT)*, helps cardiologists determine whether a patient has a significant blockage in a coronary artery. The results of this test can decrease the need for heart catheterization while still identifying those patients who may need stent placement or bypass surgery.

For this test, a patient has a CT scan. Then, specialized computer software assesses blockages so that further treatment, if needed, can be determined.

### Magnetic Resonance Imaging

Unlike other scans, which use X-ray technology, *magnetic resonance imaging (MRI)* uses powerful magnets and radio waves to produce clear, three-dimensional images of the heart's chambers and large vessels.

An MRI gives your doctor a look at your heart muscle and helps determine whether you've suffered any damage to your heart muscle from a heart attack. The test can also evaluate diseases of the larger blood vessels. Cardiac MRI may also show blood flow problems and blockages in the coronary arteries. Because MRI depends on magnetic forces, if you have a pacemaker or other metal in your body, you may not be a candidate for this test. However, some of the newer pacemakers are compatible with an MRI. Also, the special dye inserted into the blood vessels may be harmful to patients with kidney function problems.

## Cardiac Catheterization

A cardiac catheterization is performed to determine where you have blood flow problems in the heart or blockages in the coronary arteries. This test can measure blood pressure in the heart, determine how much oxygen is in the blood, and provide information about the structure and function of the heart muscle, heart valves, and arteries. Your doctor may order a cardiac catheterization if he or she suspects that you have significant CHD.

*Preparing for Cardiac Catheterization*

- Don't eat or drink anything after midnight the night before the procedure (except small amounts of water for taking medication as directed by your physician). If catheterization is scheduled for the afternoon, your doctor may allow you to have clear liquids for breakfast.

- Leave jewelry at home.

- Empty your bladder before the exam.

- Inform your doctor if you're allergic to X-ray dye. Most hospitals use the newer X-ray dyes, which decrease (but do not totally eliminate) allergic reactions. Doctors pretreat those who have dye allergies with antihistamines and corticosteroids to reduce the likelihood of an allergic reaction.

- If you're pregnant or think you might be, be sure to let your doctor know.

## Undergoing Catheterization

An intravenous line will be inserted into your arm to deliver fluids and medications. The area on your wrist or leg where the catheter will be inserted will be cleaned and prepped. *Prepping* refers to a patient's skin being cleansed with a special soap and any hair in the area is shaved. Then you'll be taken to the "cath" lab and placed on a flat table under an X-ray machine. Nurses or technologists will attach electrodes to your arms and legs, and you'll be given "twilight sedation," which will cause you to relax and sometimes fall asleep.

To perform the cardiac catheterization, the cardiologist threads a long, flexible tube, called a *catheter,* through an artery in the wrist or in the leg up into the heart. Then a liquid dye is injected. The dye shows up on an X-ray of the heart and blood vessels.

Watching the X-ray video monitor, the doctor advances the catheter through the blood vessels to your heart. During the procedure, the cardiologist may insert several catheters via the same entry site into various parts of your heart. You will not feel the catheter(s). Once they're in the heart, the catheters can perform functions such as measuring the pressure in the heart chambers, taking blood samples, and injecting X-ray dye for pictures of arteries. (This picture is called an *angiogram.*)

If you're awake when the dye is injected into the main pumping chamber of the heart or into the aorta, you'll feel a hot sensation that lasts up to twenty seconds. You may also feel your heart "skip beats." Occasionally, you may feel nauseated, but this sensation usually passes after a minute or so. These sensations are to be expected and shouldn't alarm you. However, let the doctor know when you experience these feelings. Also report any chest pain. It's important to remain very still so that the X-ray images will be clear. Most patients do not find this procedure painful.

## *If You Have a Blocked Artery*

If, at the end of a cardiac catheterization, the results show that you have a blocked artery, the cardiologist can continue on with a procedure, called *angioplasty,* or intervention to open the blockage and insert a stent that will keep the artery open. *See* chapter 9 for more details on the insertion of a stent.

## *Recovering from Cardiac Catheterization*

After the procedure is completed, the catheter will be removed. The wrist insertion site will be covered with a wristband; the pressure from the band prevents bleeding. If the cardiologist has used a leg artery to insert the catheter, he or she will often use a closure device such as a suture, plug, or sealer may to close the tiny entry point.

During this time, a nurse will monitor your vital signs and watch the catheter insertion site to make sure it's not bleeding. He or she will also monitor the pulse, color, and temperature of the wrist or leg used for the procedure. While you're in the hospital, let a nurse know if you notice any swelling, bleeding, or pain where the catheter was inserted. If your doctor used a closure device (stitches, plugs, or a type of sealer) on the insertion site, the required bed rest time is about an hour; the bed rest prevents bleeding at the insertion site.

After you've recovered sufficiently and no critical blockages are present, the doctor will release you to go home.

Before leaving the clinic or hospital, you should:

- Ask about results. You can usually talk with your doctor about your condition right after the procedure. Your doctor will likely come into the recovery room and talk with you about your results. He or she will inform any family or friends who have accompanied you to the hospital.
- Ask the doctor when you can resume eating and drinking.

- Have someone available to drive you home. You shouldn't drive for at least twenty-four hours following the procedure.

When you return home you should:

- Avoid strenuous activity for at least forty-eight hours after the procedure.

- Call the doctor's office immediately if the catheter insertion site becomes swollen, red, painful, or oozes blood, or if the limb becomes painful, cold, and pale, or has a weak or absent pulse.

- Return to the doctor's office for follow-up within five to seven days.

### Risks of Cardiac Catheterization

Cardiac catheterization is generally safe. Complications, which are rare, are more likely to occur in people who are critically ill or when catheterization is done under emergency conditions. You're also at greater risk for serious complications if you have chronic illnesses such as kidney failure, insulin-dependent diabetes, severe lung disease, severely decreased heart function, or if you're older than eighty years of age. If you have kidney problems, you're at greater risk for dye-related kidney complications. Your medical team will take special precautions to minimize any risks.

The risk is of a fatal complication, such as a heart attack, during the procedure is very low—1 in 1,000. Other potential complications include: abnormal heartbeat, puncture of a blood vessel or of the heart muscle, bleeding, blood clotting, infection at the site of the catheter insertion, or an allergic reaction to the X-ray dye.

## Coping Emotionally after a CHD Diagnosis

If your diagnostic tests indicate that you have CHD, realize that it can have an emotional impact on you. It's easy to think of CHD as a purely physical disease. However, the diagnosis of heart disease is likely to affect you emotionally. In fact, depression is a common response to the diagnosis of CHD or following a heart attack or heart surgery. It's often triggered by a sense of loss—perhaps the loss of the way your body once was or loss of your previous, familiar lifestyle. Depression may be triggered by fears—of dying, of having heart attack, or of feeling vulnerable or frail. If you find yourself unable to sleep, tearful, or having feelings of hopelessness and despair, talk with your doctor. He or she can offer treatment or referral for treatment for your symptoms of depression.

Following are some strategies for dealing with depression, anxiety, or fears about your heart disease:

*Communicate with your doctor.* Be sure to talk openly with your doctor about your condition and your emotions. If you have questions or concerns, don't wait for a scheduled appointment; call the doctor. If your doctor doesn't make him- or herself available to you, or you don't feel comfortable talking with them, find a new doctor.

*Become empowered.* By educating yourself about heart disease, making lifestyle changes, and taking your prescribed medications, you can take control of your condition rather than let it take control of you.

*Avoid denial.* Don't psychologically block out your physical problem, hoping it will "just go away."

*Don't deny your emotions.* Allow yourself your feelings. Acknowledge that having heart disease is an emotionally painful condition.

*Avoid withdrawing from friends and relatives.* Stay involved with family, friends, and colleagues.

*Talk to others.* Have a good support system. Call friends or close family members and talk about how you feel. Set yourself a goal to talk to someone about your feelings for at least a few minutes every day. Join a support group for cardiac patients. Ask your doctor for a referral to such groups.

*Get out of the house.* You may have to force yourself to go out at first, but do it. Accept invitations.

*Keep a journal.* Just writing down how you feel can help. When you've finished writing down all your negative feelings, start a new page with the heading "Things I'm Doing for Myself Today."

# 8 MEDICATIONS FOR CORONARY HEART DISEASE

After your doctor has confirmed that you have coronary heart disease, undoubtedly your next question is "What can I do about it?" Your treatment will depend on the extent of your CHD and your general health. CHD treatment aims to prevent or reverse significant artery narrowing and to protect your heart from being damaged. Medications can help.

A number of medications have proven effective in treating CHD. For many people, drug therapy can help prevent a heart attack or stroke. It can also help prevent complications and slow the progression of blockages in the arteries (atherosclerosis).

Almost all drugs, including those for CHD, have side effects—some minor, others more noticeable. For anyone taking medication, the benefits of the medication must outweigh the risks. That's why it's important that you take heart medication only under the direction of your doctor.

## Commonly Prescribed Medications

Your doctor may prescribe one or a combination of medications for you, depending on the nature of your CHD and any other health problems. The following are classes of drugs for CHD. To see a list of commonly prescribed drugs and possible side effects, see the Appendix on page 111.

## Drugs to Lower Cholesterol

If you have CHD, one of your treatment goals will be to reduce your LDL cholesterol to 100 mg/dL or less (ideally, less than 70 mg/dL). In addition to lifestyle changes, your doctor may prescribe cholesterol-lowering medications. All cholesterol-lowering medications are used to complement a heart-healthy diet and lifestyle.

A variety of drugs are available for the treatment of cholesterol and other lipid conditions. Your doctor may prescribe a combination of drugs, especially if a single cholesterol-lowering medication doesn't improve your cholesterol levels or if you cannot tolerate a drug.

### Statins

Statins are the drugs of choice for reducing cholesterol. Statins enhance the body's ability to rid itself of cholesterol. They work directly on the liver to block an enzyme that your body needs to manufacture cholesterol. The result is that cholesterol in the liver becomes depleted and cholesterol is removed from the circulating blood.

Statins are especially effective in reducing LDL cholesterol ("bad"). Some studies indicate that statins can reduce LDL cholesterol by 30 to 60 percent, usually enough to bring cholesterol levels within safe limits. Statins may also help the body reabsorb cholesterol from plaques, slowly reversing atherosclerosis. Statins have been proven to reduce the risk of a second heart attack and the risk of death from CHD. Statins are easy to take, cause few drug interactions, and have few short-term side effects. Up to 13 percent of patients may report muscle aches.

A rare side effect is a serious muscle breakdown that tends to occur when taking both a statin and a fibrate for high triglycerides. Warning signs of muscle damage would include: dark urine, muscle aches, weakness, fever, nausea, and vomiting. At the first sign of these problems, stop taking the medication immediately and contact your doctor. If caught early, problems from this uncommon side effect can be quickly and effectively treated.

Your doctor will want to periodically check your liver function because statins raise liver enzyme levels in up to 3 percent of patients. (Increase in liver enzymes may indicate inflammation or injury to the liver.) Subsequent monitoring is recommended for patients with symptoms of liver toxicity; these symptoms include fatigue, weight loss, loss of appetite, abdominal discomfort, or dark colored urine. Patients with preexisting chronic liver disease must be carefully monitored by their physicians. Do not use statins if you're pregnant.

If your doctor prescribes cholesterol-lowering medication, you will also need to:

- Follow a cholesterol-lowering diet.
- Be physically active (as recommended by your doctor).
- Lose excess weight if you're overweight.
- Stop smoking.
- Control your high blood pressure and diabetes.

Because the body makes more cholesterol at night, it is recommended that you take statins two hours after dinner or at bedtime. The drugs take four to six weeks to be effective. Avoid drinking grapefruit juice if you're taking certain statins because it can interfere with your body's ability to clear some of these drugs from the liver. Side effects also include elevation in blood sugars; however, the benefits usually outweigh any risk. Some people are allergic to statins, or they become intolerant and need other cholesterol-lowering drugs.

### PCSK9 Inhibitors

*PCSK9 inhibitors* are given by injection to lower LDL cholesterol. They are approved for those with an inherited condition called *familial hypercholesterolemia* that makes the body unable to remove LDL "bad" cholesterol from the blood. PCSK9s are also used for patients who do not get adequate results with statins or other therapies. The injections are given every two or four weeks.

These drugs have been associated with a decreased incidence of heart attack and stroke.

### Resins

Also called *bile acid resins,* these drugs can lower "bad" LDL cholesterol by about 10 to 20 percent. Even small doses of resins can lower LDL cholesterol. Resins are sometimes prescribed with a statin to increase cholesterol reduction. When these two drugs are combined, together they can lower LDL cholesterol by over 40 percent.

Resins are available in tablet and powder forms and are usually taken twice a day with meals. The powders must be mixed with water or fruit juice. Drinking large amounts of water and other liquids can help prevent gastrointestinal problems such as gas, nausea, bloating, and constipation.

### Fibrates

These drugs lower triglyceride levels by reducing the production of triglycerides and removing them from circulation. Studies have shown that fibrates can reduce triglycerides by 20 to 50 percent and increase "good" HDL cholesterol by 10 to 15 percent.

### Fish Oils

For those who have high levels of triglycerides, fish oils may help lower them. Fish oils may help reduce heart attack and stroke. The omega-3 fatty acids in fish oil cannot be made by the body; they need to come from food sources or supplements—liquid, capsules, or pills.

## Medications to Lower Blood Pressure

### Alpha-Blockers

Alpha-blockers work by relaxing muscles and helping small blood vessels remain open. These drugs keep the hormone norepinephrine from tightening the muscles in the walls of smaller arteries and veins; this action keeps vessels open, improving blood flow and lowering blood pressure. Alpha-blockers lower blood pressure by blocking the stimulation of specialized nerves.

### Beta-Blockers

Beta-blockers reduce blood pressure by decreasing heart rate, reducing the strength of the heart's contractions, and relaxing blood vessel walls. For people who have CHD and high blood pressure, a combination of beta-blockers and ACE inhibitors is generally the preferred treatment. Beta-blockers are also prescribed for other heart-related conditions. They can help normalize some types of heart rhythm disturbances (abnormal beats). They decrease the heart's need for oxygen and so are also prescribed for angina. Additionally, this medication can reduce the severity of a heart attack when given immediately; it can also decrease sudden death in people after a heart attack.

Beta-blockers may cause side effects in some people. They may cause breathlessness in people with asthma. If you have coronary spasm, beta-blockers can worsen angina. Abruptly stopping beta-blockers may cause an increase in heart rate and blood pressure. In some cases, beta-blockers worsen heart failure; however, long term, beta-blockers have been proven to improve symptoms and decrease mortality in people with heart failure.

### ACE Inhibitors

Another class of drugs, called *angiotensin-converting enzyme (ACE) inhibitors,* are effective in reducing blood pressure. These drugs block the formation of a potent chemical (angiotensin) that causes tiny arteries to constrict. The ACE inhibitors also help heal heart muscle after a heart attack; they also lower the death rate of individuals with weakened hearts. For people with diabetes, they protect kidney function.

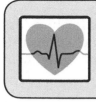 The prescription drug *Vascepa* is a type of fish oil. One study showed that it reduces the risk of heart attack and stroke by 25 percent. Along with a low-cholesterol diet, the drug decreases the amount of tryglycerides made by the body.

ACE inhibitor drugs, like other medications, have side effects. The most serious one is kidney failure in people who have narrowing of both kidney arteries. The most common side effect of ACE inhibitor drugs is a dry, hacking cough, which is reversible. These drugs can also cause some people to develop high levels of potassium in the blood; too much potassium in your blood can lead to dangerous, and possibly deadly, changes in heart rhythm. If you take an ACE inhibitor, your doctor will want to monitor your potassium blood levels and kidney function regularly.

ACE inhibitors should not be used during pregnancy; if used during pregnancy, the drug can cause low blood pressure, severe kidney failure, and excess potassium. If you're pregnant or think you might be pregnant, inform your doctor immediately.

### ARBs

*Angiotensin receptor blockers (ARBs)* are another drug that lowers blood pressure. This medication directly blocks the effects of the chemical that causes tiny arteries to constrict. These drugs are often prescribed for diabetics to protect kidney function. ARBs are also an alternative medication for people with heart attack or heart failure who cannot use ACE inhibitors. A dry cough isn't as big a problem with ARBs as it is with ACE inhibitors but still occurs in 3 to 5 percent of people.

ARBs can cause birth defects and shouldn't be taken during pregnancy.

## Diuretics

Commonly called "water pills," diuretics flush excess water and sodium (salt) from the body by increasing urination. This reduces the amount of fluid and sodium in the blood, lowering blood pressure.

## Calcium Channel Blockers

These drugs relax the blood vessels and reduce blood pressure by preventing calcium from entering the muscle cells of the heart and arteries. The drug also increases the supply of blood and oxygen to the heart while also reducing the heart's workload.

If you're taking calcium channel blockers, avoid drinking grapefruit juice at the time you take the medication. Grapefruit juice contains a component that interferes with the liver's ability to clear certain drugs, such as nifedipine *(Adalat, Procardia)*, felodipine *(Plendil)*, and nimodipine *(Nimotop)*. Drinking grapefruit juice and taking these drugs can allow toxic levels of the drugs to build up in the blood.

## Nerve Inhibitors

The sympathetic nerves extend from the brain to all parts of the body, including the arteries and their tiny branches. Nerve-inhibiting drugs reduce blood pressure by affecting control centers in the brain that keep these nerves from narrowing (constricting) blood vessels. These drugs can be very effective, but their use is limited because they cause fatigue and dry mouth.

## Vasodilators

Vasodilators reduce blood pressure by causing the muscle in the walls of the blood vessels, especially the tiny arterioles, to widen or relax. Because they may also cause the body to retain salt and water and speed heart rate, they're often prescribed in combination with diuretics and beta-blockers.

## Drugs for Angina (Chest Pain)

### Nitrates

Nitrates are often prescribed to relieve angina—pain caused by reduced blood flow to the heart. Nitrates, usually nitroglycerine, widen the coronary arteries. This increases blood flow to the heart. They also dilate the veins, which slows the return of blood to the heart and makes the heart work less.

If you have severe angina, your doctor may prescribe a *nitroglycerine (NTG)* spray or a tablet that you put under your tongue. Nitroglycerine works very fast to relieve pain. If you need daily doses of nitrate medication, your doctor may prescribe it in a capsule by mouth or as a cream or patch that's placed on the skin. Even if you take long-acting preparations (pills or patches), you may still need to take nitrate tablets or spray, as needed, if breakthrough pain occurs. Intravenous NTG is available for patients who are hospitalized.

The most problematic side effect of nitrate medication is a sudden drop in blood pressure when you stand from sitting or lying down *(orthostatic hypotension)*. If your systolic blood pressure is below 90 mmHg, nitroglycerine probably isn't a good choice. The medication can also cause headache, dizziness, rapid heartbeat, and skin flushing—feelings of warmth and rapid reddening of your neck, upper chest, or face. Some side effects, such as headache, usually lessen after taking the medication for several days. In rare cases, topical nitrates can cause a skin rash. Alcohol may worsen side effects.

*Note:* Never take nitroglycerine if you've been taking erectile dysfunction medications *Viagra, Levitra,* or *Cialis.* It can cause a life-threatening drop in blood pressure. If you've been taking one of these medications and you're having chest pain don't take nitroglycerine. Instead, go to the hospital immediately.

All forms of nitrates have a limited shelf life. Nitrates that are too old simply won't work. Talk with your pharmacist about how long your nitrates will be effective and how to store them to keep them at their peak.

### Beta-Blockers and Calcium Channel Blockers

Beta-blockers can also help relieve symptoms of angina by decreasing the heart's need for oxygen. As the name implies, calcium channel blockers block the movement of calcium in the heart, nerves, and blood vessel walls. Calcium is a mineral in the blood that can calcify in the vessel walls, causing atherosclerosis. People who aren't helped by nitroglycerine or beta-blockers can often get relief using calcium channel blockers.

## Blood Thinners

The body defends itself against bleeding by forming blood clots. However, blood's tendency to clot in the coronary arteries can also cause angina and heart attacks. There are two major ways that blood clots form:

- Platelets (tiny cells circulating in the bloodstream) stick to damaged surfaces and to one another to form a so-called white clot (white thrombus).

- Specialized blood proteins are activated and form a gel-like ball or red clot (red thrombus).

Blood thinners work to alter one or both of these blood-clotting mechanisms.

### Antiplatelet Agents

Antiplatelet drugs reduce the blood's ability to clot by inhibiting the normal functioning of platelets, cells in the blood that cause clotting. Aspirin is one of the best-known antiplatelet medications. It helps prevent blood clot formation on existing plaque, which reduces the risk of heart attacks. Over time, aspirin makes the blood more resistant to forming clots.

Aspirin is usually prescribed to all patients with CHD, unless they have an allergy or another problem. It's the first medication that's given in an emergency room during a heart attack. It's also used after coronary angioplasty and stenting to prevent blood clots and help prolong the lifespan of bypasses created during coronary bypass surgery. (*See* chapter 9 for more information on angioplasty and bypass surgery.)

### Anticoagulants

These blood-thinning drugs inhibit the specialized blood proteins that form a red blood clot (red thrombus). They are often given during and after a heart attack to prevent clots from forming. Your doctor may also prescribe an anticoagulant medication if you have atrial fibrillation (a type of irregular heartbeat) or a mechanical artificial heart valve. These drugs don't dissolve existing blood clots. They can, however, prevent new clots from forming or prevent existing clots from getting bigger. They can be administered both intravenously and by mouth.

### Thrombolytics

These drugs are used to dissolve blood clots during a heart attack. They work by increasing the blood level and action of an enzyme that breaks up blood clots. Although thrombolytics can't prevent a heart attack, they can help you survive one. To be effective, thrombolytics must be administered within the first few hours of a heart attack. They're most effective if they're given within the first hour (ideally within thirty minutes) of a patient's arrival at a hospital emergency room.

The major risk with thrombolytics is bleeding, especially bleeding into the brain. This is relatively rare (up to 1.5 percent of cases) and occurs more frequently in women over the age of seventy.

Angioplasty and stenting have replaced thrombolytics as the treatment of choice for heart attacks. These drugs are recommended for patients with heart attacks who arrive at hospitals that are not equipped to perform angioplasty and stenting and the transfer time to such a center will be excessive.

*Precautions When Taking Blood Thinners*
The following list provides guidence if you are taking blood thinners.

- Take the medication exactly as your doctor instructs.
- Ask your doctor before taking other medications or supplements, even vitamins or over-the-counter medications.
- Ask about any interactions with foods (vitamin K in broccoli and spinach) when taking warfarin.
- When taking warfarin, be sure to have blood tests regularly so your doctor can monitor how well your medications are working.
- Tell your doctor about these (and any other medications you're taking) before you have surgery.
- Let your doctor know right away if you have: red, black, or dark brown stools, heavy menstrual bleeding, or bleeding gums.

Report these conditions to your physician:

- any intense headache or stomach pain that doesn't go away
- any bouts of weakness, dizziness, fainting, or a general feeling of being unwell
- bruises or blood blisters
- pregnancy
- an accident of any kind (which could cause bleeding)

## Research Continues

In the past decade, medical science has made many new medications available for individuals with corornary heart disease. These medications have improved the quality of life and extended life for millions of patients. Meanwhile, research continues to produce even more and better drugs.

# 9 STENTS AND BYPASS SURGERY

Many people are able to control coronary heart disease with healthful lifestyle changes and medications. However, if the blockages in your coronary arteries are severe or if you continue to have frequent or disabling chest discomfort *(angina)*, you may need other treatments to improve the blood supply to your heart. Having more blood get to your heart should help reduce or eliminate angina, reduce fatigue, and possibly decrease your need for medication. These additional therapies can improve the quality and the length of your life.

One of these therapies is a procedure called *angioplasty with stent placement*. You may recall, chapter 7, Getting a Diagnosis, talked about angioplasty or heart catheterization to determine whether arteries are clogged. If an artery is blocked, a cardiologist will proceed with opening the blockage and placing a stent to prop open the blocked artery.

The second procedure is a much more extensive operation known as *coronary bypass artery graft (CABG)* surgery. Let's first examine the angioplasty and stent placement.

## Angioplasty with Stent Placement

*Angioplasty,* the procedure to place a stent, is a minimally invasive surgical procedure used to repair or unblock a blood vessel, especially a coronary artery, that has become blocked by plaque buildup. The procedure

## Stent Placement

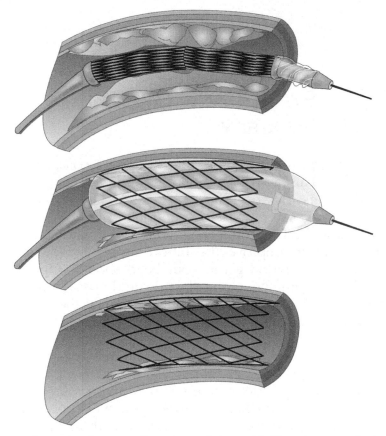

The top illustration shows a collapsed stent being guided into the artery. In the middle illustration, the balloon has opened the clogged artery. The bottom illustration shows the stent in place; the balloon has been withdrawn.

also relieves chest pain caused by a reduction in blood flow to the heart; this procedure may also minimize the risk of a heart attack.

During the procedure, a tiny balloon is used to widen the narrowed artery without the need to surgically open the chest. After the blockage is partially cleared, a stent, which is a tiny mesh tube, is inserted to keep the artery open. Stents are used in more than 95 percent of angioplasty procedures.

When stents were first introduced in the 1990s, it was soon discovered that scar tissue developed inside the stents of 20 to 35 percent of patients; this scar tissue buildup, called *restenosis* (renarrowing), created new blockages at the treatment site usually within six to twelve months after the procedure.

In an effort to eliminate an artery becoming blocked again, medical researchers developed drug-coated stents, which reduced the buildup of scar tissue and increased the likelihood that arteries will remain open. Approved by the Food and Drug Administration in 2003, these are the most popular stents used today. They have a renarrowing rate of less than 5 to 10 percent in most patients, compared to the 20 to 35 percent in patients with conventional, nonmedicated stents. Reducing the risk of renarrowing means fewer patients require another stent placement and fewer patients need bypass surgery.

## Who Is a Candidate for Stent Placement?

Previously, angioplasty with stent placement was performed only on people who had one severely blocked artery. Now, due to advances in the procedure, doctors are using angioplasty for people with multiple blockages. Studies show that the procedure provides more complete relief than medication alone for people with angina.

Depending on where the blockages are located, angioplasty is equivalent to bypass surgery in providing relief from angina, lowering risk of heart attack, and improving long-term survival rates.

Whether stent placement is right for you is a decision you and your doctor will have to make together, depending on:

- the location of your blockages
- how many blockages you have
- the extent of the blockage

- your age
- your overall health
- how well your heart is functioning
- how hardened (calcified) your plaques are
- whether you have a valve problem that would benefit from surgery

You may not be a candidate for angioplasty if:

- Your heart disease is too advanced
- The plaque is located in an area inaccessible by catheter or in an area felt to be too risky. Some locations may best be treated with bypass surgery
- The plaque is severely calcified. In the hands of a skilled interventional cardiologist, the blockage can usually be opened and treated successfully.
- Sometimes when there is complete blockage in one or more coronary arteries, especially if the artery has been blocked for a long time
- You cannot take blood-thinning medications

Still, even difficult cases may be treated. New techniques and equipment make it possible to place stents in patients who are at high risk for complications. In some cases, a heart pump that assists heart function can be used during the stent procedure. This approach may also be used for temporary support when heart function is weak.

## Undergoing a Stent Procedure

Angioplasty and stenting are typically performed in a catheterization suite or "cath lab" in a hospital. Patients are given local anesthesia and sedation with a relaxant medication similar to Valium.

The procedure takes thirty minutes to two hours, depending on the extent of blockages. In most cases, it requires at most an overnight hospital stay.

First, the cardiologist will numb the area in which an incision will be made; then he or she will make a small

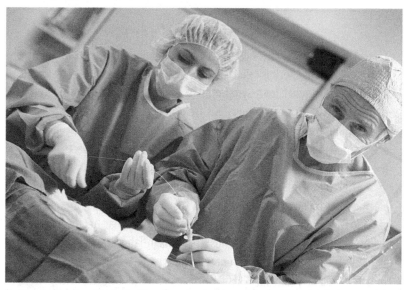

During a heart catheterization (angiogram), a thin guide wire is inserted in a blood vessel in the wrist or the groin; from there, the tube is maneuvered through the vessel and into the heart. Dye is injected and X-rays are taken. The dye helps doctors detect blockages.

incision in one of two places—either in the wrist or in the groin—to access an artery. Next, using X-ray technology and a television monitor as a guide, the physician will thread a long, narrow tube, called a *guide catheter,* through the artery to the heart. where the blockage is occurring. The cardiologist will inject a small amount of X-ray dye. This dye will enable the cardiologist to see the exact location of the blockage.

### Stent Insertion

After the guiding catheter is placed, a second, smaller catheter equipped with a deflated balloon is inserted into the guide catheter. After the wire is threaded across the blockage, the balloon is inflated to widen the blocked artery. Then, a wire-mesh stent is placed to keep the artery open.

---

**Non-Surgical Treatment for Angina**

For those who are not candidates for angioplasty, an alternative treatment is available. It is called *enhanced external counter pulsation (EECP)*, and it provides relief from symptoms of angina. It may be considered in combination with medications. The treatments, usually administered as a series, aim for long-lasting improvement in blood flow, which increases exercise tolerance. Some people have experienced positive effects for up to five years following treatment.

The treatment, which isn't painful but can be uncomfortable, involves placing long inflatable cuffs (similar to blood pressure cuffs) around each of your legs while you're lying down. As each heartbeat begins, the cuffs deflate, and as each heartbeat ends, the cuffs inflate. This "milking" action increases blood flow into the coronary arteries while reducing the amount of work required by your heart. EECP consists of a series of treatments, one to two hours a day, five days per week, for a total of thirty-five hours.

---

During this part of the procedure, you may feel chest pain or pressure, which is similar to the discomfort you may have experienced prior to the procedure. That's because while the balloon is inflated, blood flow through the artery is temporarily blocked. Let the doctor know if you feel pain. In most cases, the pain goes away once the balloon is deflated.

After the balloon catheter is removed, X-rays are taken to see how well blood is flowing through the affected artery. If blood is flowing well, the guide catheter will be removed.

At this point, if your procedure was performed through the artery in your wrist, you'll have a special wristband put on that will put pressure on the tiny incision to prevent bleeding. You will be able to move as soon as the procedure is completed. If the catheter was inserted through your groin, the tiny incision may be closed with a suture or plug. You will not be allowed to move for several hours; this prevents bleeding at the entry point.

### Recovery from Stent Placement

The medical team will monitor you for six to twenty-four hours. Be sure to let the nurses or doctor know if you feel any pain or discomfort following your angioplasty procedure.

You'll need to return to your doctor within a couple of weeks and then within six months; at that time, your physician will evaluate how well the procedure is keeping your artery open. The follow-up, which involves a checkup, ECG, or stress tests, can be done in your doctor's office. These procedures are noninvasive and painless. If a stress test indicates it's safe, your doctor may recommend a *cardiac rehabilitation program*—a structured plan of education, exercise, and other lifestyle changes to reduce your cardiac risk factors.

### Keeping Stents Open

Patients with newly placed stents are prescribed aspirin to be taken indefinitely along with a blood-thinning drug. These drugs, Plavix, Brilinta, or Effient, are taken for up to twelve months after receiving a stent. However, some patients who are at high risk for clots are treated for a longer period, and those at high risk for bleeding may be considered for a shorter period—as little as three months.

It is important that you and your cardiologist discuss the risks of a stented artery renarrowing, risk of blood clots, or bleeding.

## How Effective Is Stenting?

Nearly 2 million angioplasty/stent procedures are performed in the United States every year. The success rate for treating arteries that are not totally blocked exceed 95 percent. The success of treating total blockages with angioplasty depends largely on how long the artery has

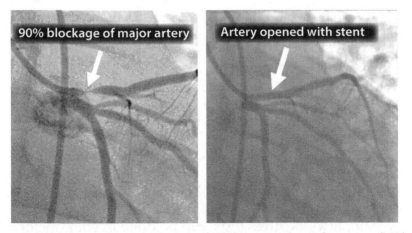

At left, the photo shows narrowing in the left anterior descending artery (LAD). The photo on the right shows the same artery after placement of a stent.

been totally blocked. If the artery has been completely blocked for less than three months, the angioplasty success rate is above 80 percent. It drops to less than 50 percent if the artery has been completely blocked for more than three months. For many people, the procedure relieves angina better than medication alone.

Angioplasty/stenting is easier for the patient and less invasive than coronary artery bypass graft surgery (CABG), which is discussed later in this chapter. Receiving a stent doesn't involve general anesthesia, hospital stays are shorter, and recovery time is faster. Major complications are unusual. If the procedure needs to be repeated, the risks are no higher than the initial procedure, whereas a repeat bypass operation carries higher risk than the first. This risk, however, depends on the distribution of the blockage(s).

## How Safe Is Stent Placement?

As mentioned in an earlier chapter, the angioplasty procedure is relatively safe. Less than 1 percent of patients who undergo angioplasty will need emergency bypass surgery during the procedure. There is a 1 percent risk of death from undergoing an angioplasty procedure. The risk of having a minor heart attack during the procedure is 2 to 6 percent, a major heart attack less than 1 percent.

The incidence of heart attack, stroke, and death following angioplasty is higher for women than for men. This may be because women who undergo the procedure tend to be older and have a higher incidence of high blood pressure, diabetes, high blood cholesterol, and other health problems than men who undergo the procedure.

In addition to the rare risks of heart attack, stroke, and death, other complications may occur. These complications are usually treatable. They include:

- injury or puncture of the artery during insertion of the catheter

- increased risk of clot formation inside the artery

- blockages made worse if the angioplasty causes scar tissue to form, creating greater blockage

Your physician must advise you of the risk of not treating your CHD blockages weighed against the risk of complications.

## Coronary Artery Bypass Graft Surgery

Although angioplasty is an effective treatment for many, it's not always the best treatment for everyone. Some individuals may require *coronary artery bypass graft surgery (CABG)*, pronounced "cabbage." This is also referred to as *open heart surgery*. This is a major surgical procedure performed to increase blood supply to the heart. The bypass procedure involves taking a piece of a blood vessel, from the chest and/or leg, and stitching it onto the blocked artery in order to replenish blood supply. In many cases, more than one artery is blocked, requiring multiple bypasses.

Those who may need bypass surgery include people whose arteries are chronically totally blocked, who have narrowing in all the coronary arteries, or who have

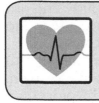 In some patients, bypass surgery lowers the risk of heart attack and other health problems. It is the most common type of open-heart surgery in the United States. Most people have excellent results and live symptom-free.

narrowing in the left main coronary artery. Also, people who are diabetic and have narrowing in the artery that supplies the front of the heart (left anterior descending artery or LAD) generally have better results with bypass surgery, especially if the narrowings involves a long segment of the arteries.

## Who Is a Candidate for Bypass Surgery?

In general, bypass surgery is used when coronary blockages are severe and widespread, especially if three arteries are blocked or the blockages occur at critical locations in the heart's circulatory system. Because bypass is a major operation, your doctor will recommend it only after careful consideration of the location and extent of your blockages. Other factors include the overall health of your heart, your age, and other non-heart health problems you may have.

You may be a candidate for bypass surgery if:

- Your angina is debilitating and interferes with normal functions of daily life.

- Two or all three main coronary arteries are narrowed 75 percent or more. (Some people with CHD in only one vessel may also benefit.)

- The left main coronary artery is 70 percent or more narrowed (50 percent in some cases).

- You have poor function of the left ventricle, the heart's main pumping station, which may improve with a renewed blood supply.

- You have a very abnormal exercise or nuclear test despite the absence of symptoms.

## Bypass Grafts

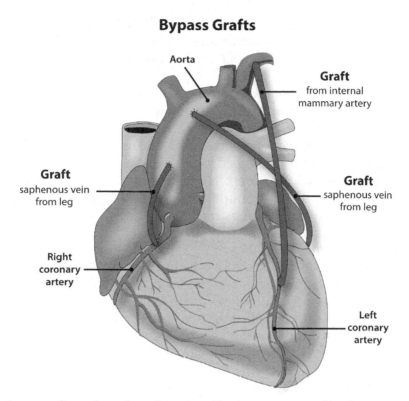

Bypass grafts are shown here. Using magnification, surgeons use hair-fine sutures to attach the grafts.

- You're not a good candidate for angioplasty/ stenting.
- You've already undergone a catheter treatment that's been unsuccessful.
- Bypasses from a previous operation have closed.

## Undergoing Bypass Graft Surgery

*Preparing for Surgery*

The night before your surgery, you'll shower with a special soap to decrease the risk of infection. Your doctor will give you instructions on what medications you can take prior to surgery. Your doctor will likely ask you to not take blood-thinning medications (except aspirin) to avoid the risk of bleeding during and immediately following the surgery.

A nurse will prepare you for surgery by prepping your chest and legs (remember, a vein may be removed from your leg). About an hour before surgery, you'll be given a sedative to help you relax. After you're in the operating room, the anesthesiologist will give you a general anesthetic to put you to sleep. He or she will insert a special intravenous line to monitor your blood pressure and the pressure inside your lungs during the operation.

### Undergoing the Procedure

The procedure takes two to five hours, depending on the number of bypasses and the complexity of the surgery. To begin the operation, your surgeon will expose your heart by making a vertical incision through the middle of the chest and through the breastbone. After the heart is exposed, you may be put on the heart-lung bypass, or pump oxygenator.

Specialized health professionals called *perfusionists* operate this machine. The heart-lung machine oxygenates the blood like the lungs would. Then it pumps the blood into the aorta downstream from the heart, where it flows to all the organs. While you're on the heart-lung bypass, your heart is stopped and blood doesn't flow to it. This allows the surgeon to work with precision on the heart while it's not moving. Patients remain on the heart-lung machine only as long as it takes to complete the procedure. Then, the heart is restarted.

### Harvesting Blood Vessels

After the chest is opened, one or more vessels will be "harvested." In more than 90 percent of cases, a vessel inside the chest wall is used; the vessel is called the *internal mammary artery*. The body has two such

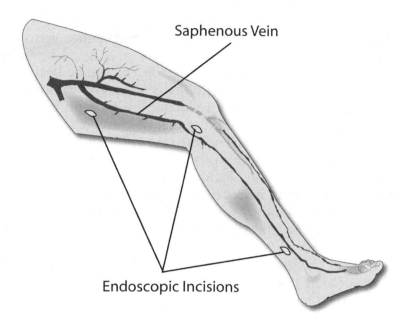

**Saphenous Vein**

**Endoscopic Incisions**

When additional veins are needed for bypass surgery, the saphenous vein, which runs down the inside of the leg, is often used.

mammary arteries—one on the left (LIMA) and one on the right side (RIMA) of the chest. The right mammary artery is used less often in bypass. The mammary arteries tend to stay open longer than other blood vessels that can be used. When a mammary artery is used, the surgeon usually doesn't have to entirely remove it. Instead, he or she reconnects the downstream part of the mammary artery to the coronary artery, bypassing the blockage.

Sometimes, a vein from a leg is used. Many people are concerned about having a blood vessel taken from their leg for the bypass operation. Removal of a vessel will not affect the health of your leg. The arteries or veins used in bypass aren't essential. Removing, or "harvesting," them doesn't significantly impact the blood flow from where they're taken.

If a vein from a leg is used, most bypasses use a vein that runs down the inside of the leg. Sometimes veins are taken from both legs. A surgeon or a surgical assistant will make an incision on the inside of one or both legs to remove the vein(s). Minimally invasive endoscopic techniques are now used, reducing the incision length to a few inches and lowering the risk of complications.

After a leg vein is removed, one end of it is connected to the aorta and the other to the coronary artery downstream from the blockage. In some cases, veins may be taken from the backs of the legs or arms, or an artery that supplies blood to the hand may be used. If needed, an artery in the abdomen can be redirected and used as a bypass graft.

After the grafts are in place, the heart is "rewarmed." The surgeon uses electric shock to restart the heart and then closes incisions.

### Recovery in Hospital

After surgery, you'll be taken to a cardiac surgery recovery room or intensive care unit for twenty-four to thirty-six hours. Small tubes that have been placed in your chest and arms will remain in place for twenty-four hours. These tubes allow medical staff to check for internal bleeding, give drugs and fluids, withdraw blood samples, drain fluid, and continuously monitor your blood pressure.

Small electrodes on your chest let the medical staff monitor your heart's rate and rhythm with an ECG. A breathing tube that goes through your mouth into your windpipe, which helps you breathe during surgery, is usually removed within the first twenty-four hours.

After the first twenty-four hours following surgery, recovery is usually fairly quick. You should be alert and able to eat and walk. If you've had one or more veins removed from your legs, you may need to wear elastic support stockings to help circulation and reduce swelling.

About 20 percent of people who undergo bypass surgery require a blood transfusion following surgery. Thirty to forty percent develop erratic heart rhythm problems (atrial fibrillation) that require special care, but these are easily treated in most cases. A few patients develop infection at the wound site. Barring these complications, you should be able to leave the hospital in four to six days.

### Potential Complications

Today, 95 percent of individuals who undergo coronary bypass surgery will not have serious complications. But complications are possible. These include:

- bleeding from incision site
- heart rhythm problems
- blood clots
- chest pain
- infection of the chest incision
- kidney problems
- low-grade fever
- pneumonia
- memory loss, which often improves after a few months
- heart attack or stroke, if a blood clot breaks loose after surgery
- failure of the bypass graft

The risk of death as a result of bypass surgery is very low—between 1 and 2 percent. The risk of death for women is twice the risk for men; one reason for this is women often do not seek treatment until their heart disease is more advanced.

If you must undergo the surgery during an emergency situation such as a heart attack, your risk of dying increases to 5 to 8 percent. Fortunately, emergency surgery is less common than it was prior to the availability of stents. The risks are also higher for people who are older or who have extensive scarring from previous heart attacks.

Surgeons at hospitals where they commonly perform bypass surgeries generally have superior outcomes.

### Recovery at Home

You'll need to see your doctor in a week or so to have any external stitches or staples removed from your chest; most of the time the stitches are under the skin and don't need to be removed. If you have stitches in your leg, they'll need to stay in a few days longer. Most people receive absorbable stitches that are placed under the skin and they disappear on their own.

Your surgery incisions should heal within about six weeks. If you have a sedentary job, you'll likely be able to return to work in about four weeks. If you have a physically demanding occupation, you may need to wait six weeks or longer. Your doctor will usually recommend a monitored exercise program. You may participate in the program while you are working in a light job. However, if you have a job requiring heavy physical labor, you'll probably need to complete the monitored exercise program before returning to work.

During your recovery period, it's important to avoid heavy lifting and take time to build up your endurance. You can't drive for six weeks. At first, you'll likely feel weak and tired. That's understandable, considering that a week in bed shrinks muscle strength by 15 percent.

It takes a lot of energy for your body to heal itself. Walking is a good way to regain your strength and energy. You'll want to keep an eye out for warning signs of infection, fluid retention, or problems with your bypass, including:

- redness or drainage at the incision site
- fever
- chills

- increasing fatigue
- weight gain over five pounds in a few days
- changes in heart rate or rhythms (palpitations or skipped beats)
- swollen ankles (Often the leg from which the vein was taken swells more, making the legs feel unequal.)

## Long-Term Results

Coronary artery bypass substantially improves symptoms in 90 percent of those who undergo the operation. However, sometimes narrowing develops in the bypass vessels themselves. Ten years after surgery, one-third of venous bypasses (vein from leg) are closed, one-third are narrowed, and one-third remain wide open. The results with mammary artery bypasses (artery from chest) are better—more than 96 percent remain open after ten years.

On average, the five-year survival rate for men who have undergone bypass is 90 to 94 percent. For women, the five-year survival rate is 87 to 91 percent. (A five-year survival rate refers to the likelihood that an individual will be alive at least five years later.) Results are improved when patients are continued on aspirin and statins.

## 10 MAKING LIFESTYLE CHANGES

Medical science has made great strides in treating coronary heart disease (CHD). New and better medications are more effective and have fewer side effects. Surgical treatments are more sophisticated than ever, leading to fewer complications and better outcomes. However, leading heart organizations, including the National Heart, Lung, and Blood Institute, agree that changing unhealthful lifestyle habits is still the single most important thing you can do to stop heart disease from progressing.

There's evidence that lifestyle changes such as diet, exercise, and learning to handle stress may prevent a heart attack and may even reverse the narrowing of arteries.

### Develop a Good Nutrition Plan

Adopting a healthier lifestyle means changing your habits not only in the way you eat, but in your attitude about food. Since you've acquired these habits over a lifetime, it will take some time to change them. Basic tips for good nutrition include:

- Make sure your diet is balanced and that you eat a wide variety of foods daily.
- Eat high-fiber foods, including fruits, vegetables, whole grains, and beans.
- Limit fat, sugar, and salt in your diet. When it comes to heart health, controlling cholesterol levels is crucial.

## Control Cholesterol Intake

Our bodies need some fat to support cell development. However, as stated earlier, there are "good" fats and "bad" fats. The National Cholesterol Education Program (NCEP) helps us understand the types of fats in our food and provides guidelines for which ones to avoid and which ones to include in our diets.

### Eat Less Saturated Fat

Saturated fats contribute to increased LDL ("bad") cholesterol levels and can increase your risk of coronary heart disease. These fats are found in dairy products, fatty meats, poultry skin, some commercially prepared baked goods, and tropical oils such as coconut, palm, and palm kernel. NCEP guidelines for saturated fat intake are less than 7 percent of total calories; this can help reduce LDL cholesterol by 8 to 10 percent.

### Avoid Trans Fats

Trans fats are also known to increase LDL ("bad") cholesterol and decrease the protective HDL ("good") cholesterol. They can increase your risk of CHD. Trans fats are often found in fast foods, commercial baked products, snack foods, fried foods, certain margarines, and shortening.

Trans fats are formed by the process of changing unsaturated oils into trans fats, which are solid at room temperature. This process, known as *hydrogenation,* is used by the food industry because trans fats increase product shelf life and improve taste in certain foods. Select food products that say "No trans fats" and avoid foods that include the words "hydrogenated" or "partially hydrogenated" on their labels. Consume as few trans fats as possible. It's best to avoid them completely.

## Choose Polyunsaturated Fats

Include polyunsaturated fats in your diet instead of saturated fats. Polyunsaturated fats are known to reduce LDL cholesterol. They are liquid at both room temperature and in the refrigerator. They are found in margarines, salad dressings, mayonnaise, vegetable oils (sunflower, safflower, soybean, cottonseed, and corn), nuts, sunflower seeds, and pumpkin seeds. Experts recommend consuming up to 10 percent of daily calories of polyunsaturated fats; more than this amount may decrease your HDL cholesterol.

## Add Omega-3 Fats to Your Diet

The omega-3 fats are another type of polyunsaturated fat that may help lower the risk of heart disease and stroke; they do this by helping to maintain a regular heartbeat, lower triglycerides and inflammation, and relax artery walls. The best sources of omega-3 fats are fatty fish such as salmon, mackerel, herring, trout, and sardines. Other sources include canola, flax, soybean, and walnut oils; walnuts; ground flaxseeds; and omega-3 eggs. Omega-3 fats may also be found in certain dairy products and margarines.

Studies have shown that having at least two servings of fatty fish per week may greatly reduce the risk of dying from CHD or stroke. If you aren't able to get fish oil from your diet, try incorporating the oils and nuts listed above more often. Fish-oil supplements may be beneficial, but it's important to speak with your doctor before starting to take them.

## Choose Monounsaturated Fats

Monounsaturated fats are another kind of fat that you should include in your diet rather than saturated fats. Like polyunsaturated fats, monounsaturated fats are known to decrease LDL cholesterol. Also, they do not lower the protective action of the good cholesterol—HDL. These fats are found in oils such as olive, peanut, and

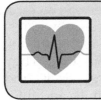

**Heart Notes**

Every calorie counts. Eating only 50 excess calories per day results in 5 pounds of weight gain a year.

canola; in some nut butters; and in peanuts, almonds, pumpkin seeds, flaxseeds, sunflower seeds, avocados, some nonhydrogenated margarines, and olives. The NCEP recommends that you consume up to 20 percent of your total daily calories come from this type of fat.

### Watch Your Total Fat Intake

Fat in the diet is necessary to absorb the fat-soluble vitamins A, D, E, and K, which we need for energy and important bodily functions. However, too much fat in your diet contributes to overweight or obesity, which will increase your risk for CHD and other medical conditions. It's important to focus on getting fat in your diet from monounsaturated and polyunsaturated fat sources. Make total fat intake 25 to 30 percent of your diet.

### Limit Intake of Dietary Cholesterol

Not to be confused with your blood cholesterol, dietary cholesterol comes from animal products, such as meats, egg yolks, shellfish, organ meats, and high-fat dairy products.

In general, the cholesterol that you get from food does not have a strong influence on your blood cholesterol, but if you are at a higher risk of CHD, the cholesterol that you get from food may raise your LDL cholesterol level. The NCEP recommends that you have no more than 200 milligrams of cholesterol daily from your diet; this can decrease LDL cholesterol by 3 to 5 percent.

## Choose the Right Carbohydrates

Get 50 to 60 percent of your diet from carbohydrates, but be selective. Carbohydrates consist of starches, sugars, and fiber and are an important part of your diet. They supply us with vitamins, minerals, and energy. Fruits and vegetables, whole grains, fat-free or low-fat milk and milk products or soy beverages, and legumes are excellent choices. Limit your intake of refined grains such as white bread, white pasta, and white rice.

A diet that contains more than 60 percent carbohydrates can raise your triglycerides and lower your protective HDL cholesterol, which can increase your risk for CHD.

## Increase Your Intake of Fiber

Fiber, also called *roughage,* is an important part of a healthful diet. Nutritious foods such as fresh fruits, vegetables, oats and other grains, beans, nuts, and seeds are high in fiber. Fiber can help you lower your risk of heart disease, manage your blood glucose levels, and lose weight.

Foods high in fiber are digested more slowly and so reduce the rate at which your body releases sugars into your bloodstream. Fiber helps lower your blood pressure and may help reduce your overall cholesterol. It also helps stabilize blood sugar levels. Fiber helps make you feel full. Most Americans eat less than half of the fiber they should be getting. It's recommended that you eat 20 to 30 grams of fiber daily.

## Include Heart-Healthy Proteins in Your Diet

Protein comes from both animal and vegetable sources. Animal sources include beef, chicken, pork, veal, eggs, and cheese. Vegetable sources include tofu (made from soybeans), textured vegetable protein, and foods containing soy, legumes, nuts, and seeds. Choosing lean animal protein sources and at least two servings of vegetable protein sources per day can help to decrease LDL cholesterol levels. The NCEP recommends that protein intake make up 20 percent of your diet.

## Reduce Salt Intake

Sodium, or salt, is abundant in the North American diet and it can increase blood pressure. The Dietary Guidelines for Americans recommends reducing your sodium intake to less than 2,300 milligrams daily, which is equivalent to one teaspoon of salt. If you're over fifty; have high blood pressure, diabetes, or chronic kidney disease; or are African American, these guidelines recommend reducing sodium intake to 1,500 milligrams daily. You can decrease your sodium intake by removing the saltshaker from your table and flavoring your foods with herbs, spices, lemon juice, garlic, and vinegar.

Processed foods are often loaded with sodium. Fast-food items are often very high in sodium. If you dine out often, you're probably having a lot more sodium in your diet than you should.

## Follow the DASH Eating Plan

*DASH* stands for Dietary Approaches to Stop Hypertension. Studies have shown that following the nutrient-rich DASH Eating Plan can help with hypertension or blood pressure control. There's an added benefit—the plan also helps improve your cholesterol levels. The goal is to follow a healthful eating plan that is low in saturated and total fat and dietary cholesterol; the plan should include fruits, vegetables, and fat-free (or low-fat) milk and milk products.

Also included are fish, poultry, nuts, and whole grains. The potassium, magnesium, and calcium from these foods help reduce blood pressure. (Ask your doctor about having magnesium and calcium in your diet.) Also, in the DASH Plan, intake of sugars from food and beverages and red meat is reduced. The addition of other lifestyle changes contributes to further blood pressure reduction.

103

## Body Mass Index

| Body Mass Index (BMI) | Classification | Risk of developing health problems |
|---|---|---|
| Less than 18.5 | Underweight | Increased |
| 18.5–24.9 | Normal weight | Lowered |
| 25.0–29.9 | Overweight | Increased |
| 30.0–34.9 | Obese Class I | High |
| 35.0–39.9 | Obese Class II | Very high |
| Greater than 40.0 | Obese Class III | Extremely high |

To determine your BMI classification, see the BMI chart in the Appendix on page 117..

These dietary strategies work well, but continue taking your blood pressure medication if it's been prescribed. It's important to note that salt substitutes may be harmful to people who have certain diseases and conditions. If you are considering using them, it's recommended to speak with your doctor first.

## Manage Your Weight

According to the Centers for Disease Control and Prevention, nearly two-thirds of Americans are either overweight or obese. Being overweight can increase your risk of heart disease, stroke, diabetes, certain cancers, and other medical conditions and diseases.

A weight loss of 5 to 10 percent can improve your blood fats, blood pressure, and blood sugar control. The NCEP recommends a gradual weight loss of one half to one pound per week and a 10 percent weight loss over six months, which can decrease LDL cholesterol by 5 to 8 percent.

*Body Mass Index (BMI)* is a measure of your weight in relation to your height. The higher your BMI, the greater your risk is of developing health problems. *See* the chart above and the BMI chart in the Appendix to determine your BMI.

## Beware of Fad Diets

Weight management is a process that requires a strong foundation of healthful eating habits over the long term. Remember, when it comes to weight loss, if a weight-loss program sounds too good to be true, it probably *is* too good to be true. In addition, these diets may be harmful from a nutrition point of view and they set you up for disappointment and frustration.

## Choosing a Weight-Loss Program

Your doctor or a registered dietitian can help you with a healthy weight-loss plan. Here are some helpful tips to remember.

- Start the day with a well-balanced breakfast.
- Eat at regular times, having three balanced meals daily.
- Make snacks healthful with foods such as vegetables and fruits, low-fat dairy products, and whole grains.
- Choose foods and beverages that are lower in sugar and fat.
- Prepare foods with little or no fat by steaming, baking, broiling, stir-frying, grilling, sautéing, or barbecuing.
- Create a grocery shopping list and do not go to the grocery store hungry.
- Keep a food diary. You may be surprised by how much you are actually eating. This may also help you follow a healthy eating plan.
- Pay attention to feelings of hunger. Emotions often affect how we eat.
- Watch portion sizes. Using smaller plates and glasses can be helpful. Save the second helpings for vegetables.

- Eat slowly. It typically takes about fifteen to twenty minutes for your brain to let you know that you are full.

- Consult the U.S. Department of Agriculture's website to learn about eating the right amount of foods from each food group. Visit www.choosemyplate.gov.

- Total your daily calorie count. If you take in more calories than your body needs, you will gain weight. This can contribute to increasing your risk of CHD, stroke, high blood pressure, diabetes, joint conditions, and certain cancers. It's important to remember that having too much "healthy" food can also raise your weight. Meet your nutritional requirements without exceeding your energy needs. It's all about balance.

## Lower Your Blood Pressure

Nearly one in four Americans has *high blood pressure (HBP)*. Also called *hypertension,* HBP occurs when small arteries (arterioles) become constricted, which makes it difficult for blood to pass through them. This forces the heart to work harder, straining both the heart and the arteries. As the heart works harder, over time, it can enlarge. If the heart becomes sufficiently enlarged, it may be unable to pump enough blood throughout the body (a condition called *heart failure*). Organs denied the blood and oxygen they need can't work properly. HBP can also cause the arteries and arterioles to become scarred and less elastic, leading to atherosclerosis.

You can't do anything about your gender, family history, age, race, or preexisting health conditions, all of which can influence your blood pressure. However, you can make these changes to lower your blood pressure:

- Lose excess weight.
- Limit alcohol to one to two drinks daily.

- Exercise regularly.
- Limit salt intake.
- Get enough potassium, calcium, and magnesium.

## Stop Smoking

Quitting smoking is one of the most important things you can do for your heart and for your overall health. Smoking causes more than 400,000 deaths per year in this country. It's a major cause of CHD and heart attack. Smoking causes as many as 30 percent of the CHD-related deaths in the United States each year. Smoking magnifies other CHD risk factors, increasing the risk. In fact, if you smoke, you're two to six times more likely to have a heart attack compared with nonsmokers. Smokers who have heart attacks are more likely to die than nonsmokers. The following list details the negative effects of smoking:

- reduces the ability of the blood to carry oxygen
- raises "bad" LDL cholesterol
- decreases "good" HDL cholesterol
- damages the lining of the coronary arteries, making them more vulnerable to plaque
- makes the blood coagulate more easily, increasing the risk of blood clots
- may trigger coronary spasm
- may lead to irregular heart rhythms

In addition, cigarette smoking is the biggest risk for *peripheral vascular disease*—narrowing of the blood vessels in the arms and legs. It also increases the risk for several types of cancer, chronic lung diseases, asthma, infertility, and impotence. Quitting smoking can dramatically lower your risk for heart disease and other health problems, no matter how long you've smoked. The risk to your heart drops soon after you quit. Within two years of quitting smoking, your chances of dying from a heart attack will be cut in half. In ten years, your risk will be nearly the same as for someone who has never smoked, depending on your other risk factors.

## Exercise Regularly

The benefits of regular exercise are many. Not only does exercise decrease your risk of coronary heart disease, it helps to decrease "bad" LDL cholesterol and triglycerides and increase "good" HDL cholesterol. Exercise also decreases blood pressure, improves blood sugar control, and increases flexibility and muscle strength.

Other benefits of exercise include improved respiratory functioning, decreased risk of bone loss and osteoporosis, reduced fatigue, and increased energy. As mentioned earlier, stress is a risk factor for heart disease and being physically active can be very helpful in reducing stress. Not only does exercise enhance physical health, it also helps you feel better emotionally. Exercise has been proven to decrease anxiety, anger, depression, and even improve concentration and overall brain functioning. Exercise also can help raise people's self-esteem by improving their body image.

It is recommended that adults aim for a minimum of 150 minutes of moderate-intensity activity each week. Or, strive weekly for 75 minutes of vigorous-intensity aerobic physical activity. Benefits from aerobic activity can be achieved with at least ten minutes of exercise at a time, spread out during the week. Focusing on muscle-strengthening exercises two or more days during the week will provide additional health benefits. Find activities that you will enjoy, such as walking, swimming, cycling, and dancing. It's recommended that you speak with your doctor before starting an exercise program.

## Set Goals for Success

To begin an exercise program, start slowly and gradually increase your activity level. Research clearly points out that your chances of continuing and succeeding with an exercise regimen increase significantly if you set goals. You might find it helpful to use the S.M.A.R.T guidelines for setting exercise and weight-loss goals. The guidelines are as follows:

**S:** *Specific.* Keep goals specific. For example, you may want to set a goal to lose ten pounds rather than say, "I want to lose weight."

**M:** *Measurable.* Keep goals measurable. Keep track of your exercise sessions so you can measure your progress.

**A:** *Attainable.* Set goals that are attainable. Keep them simple and practical.

**R:** *Realistic.* Keep goals realistic. Don't try to make up for years of inactivity in a short amount of time.

**T:** *Timely.* Set a time or date for reaching your goal. Without a goal date, your chances for success decrease.

Finally, exercise should not be used as a quick fix along with a crash diet to lose weight. It is not something to be picked up for a while and then dropped when it becomes inconvenient. Rather, exercise needs to be a personal commitment spanning your entire life. Is anything really more important than improving your health and your quality of life? Increasing your physical activity is one of the most precious gifts you can give yourself and those you love.

## Reduce Stress

Do stress and certain personality traits cause CHD and subsequent heart attacks? This question is still being hotly debated. Much of the research indicates that one's response to stress and the traits of hard-driving personality types (so-called "type As") can increase the risk of heart disease. We don't know if it's how stress influences the body directly or whether it's the unhealthy responses to it (smoking, overeating, drinking, inactivity)—or a combination—that increases CHD risk. Whatever the cause, doctors do know that psychological stress can trigger:

- increases in blood pressure
- rapid heart rate
- narrowing of arteries
- chest pain
- activation of clotting agents in the blood
- release of fats into the bloodstream
- release of the hormone cortisol, which raises blood cholesterol
- dangerous heart rhythm disturbances (arrhythmias)

What exactly is *stress?* It's a term used to describe one's response to physical, emotional, and environmental factors. It's not the events or situations that cause stress. It's our reaction to them. All of us know people who just seem to serenely go through life. Nothing ever seems to bother them. Then there are others who react—or overreact—to the least little inconvenience or disappointment with anger, hostility, worry, anxiety, depression, and other unhealthy emotions.

One study published in the journal *Circulation* found that people who frequently feel depressed are more likely to develop heart disease. Another found the risk of heart attack increases for at least two hours following an angry outburst. Still other studies suggest that a chronic state of stress can cause permanent increases in heart rate, blood pressure, and possibly blood cholesterol, all of which increase the risk of CHD and heart attack.

Most heart experts recommend a program of stress management as a part of an overall treatment plan for CHD. Look for ways to decrease the stress in your life. Basic tips include: learn to let your body relax, eliminate stressful situations in your life, exercise, and get plenty of rest.

# APPENDIX

## Commonly Prescribed Drugs for CHD

### Drugs to Lower Cholesterol

### Statins

atorvastatin *(Lipitor)*
fluvastatin *(Lescol)*
lovastatin *(Mevacor)*
pitavastatin *(Livalo)*
pravastatin *(Pravachol)*
rosuvastatin *(Crestor)*
simvastatin *(Zocor)*

*Side effects:* headache, difficulty sleeping, flushing of the skin, muscle aches, tenderness or weakness, drowsiness, dizziness, nausea or vomiting, abdominal cramping or pain.

### PCSK9 Inhibitors

alirocumab *(Praluent)*
evolocumab *(Repatha)*

*Side effects:* headache, constipation, rash, nausea, flushing, edema (fluid build-up in tissues), drowsiness, and low blood pressure.

### Cholesterol-Absorption Inhibitor

ezetimibe *(Zetia)*

*Side effects:* diarrhea, back pain, stomach or abdominal pain, numbness or tingly feeling, tired feeling, headache, dizziness, depressed mood.

111

## Resins

cholestyramine *(Questran)*
colestipol *(Colestid)*
colesevelam *(WelChol)*

*Side effects:* bloating, stomach upset, constipation, vomiting, diarrhea, loss of appetite.

## Drugs to Lower Triglycerides

### Fibrates

fenofibrate *(Tricor, Triglide)*
fenofibric acid *(Trilipix)*
gemfibrozil *(Lopid)*

*Side effects:* stomach pain, nausea, vomiting, unusual muscle pain, tenderness, weakness, yellowing of eyes or skin, dark urine.

### Fish Oils

omega-3 fish oil *(Vascepa EPA: eicosapentaenoic acid)*
omega fish oil *(Epanova: DHA and EPA)*
omega fish oil and EPA *(Lovaza DHA: docosahexaenoic acid and EPA)*

*Side effects:* joint pain, sore throat, indigestion, bruising, elevated liver tests, burping, indigestion, constipation.

## Drugs to Lower Blood Pressure

### Alpha-Blockers

doxazosin mesylate *(Cardura)*
prazosin hydrochloride *(Minipress)*
terazosin hydrochloride *(Hytrin)*

*Side effects:* sudden drops in blood pressure when sitting up or standing up, headaches, nausea, swollen legs or ankles, tiredness, weakness or feeling lethargic, sleep disturbance, tremor, rash or itchiness of the skin, rarely, they may cause problems with erections in men.

### Beta-Blockers

atenolol *(Tenormin)*
bisoprolol *(Zebeta)*

112

**Beta-Blockers (Continued)**
carvedilol *(Coreg)*
metoprolol *(Lopressor, Toprol XL)*
nadolol *(Corgard)*
nebivolol *(Bystolic)*
propranolol *(Inderal)*
timolol *(Blocadren)*

*Side effects:* dizziness, weakness, drowsiness or fatigue, cold hands and feet, dry mouth, skin, or eyes, headache, upset stomach, diarrhea or constipation.

**Combination Beta-Blocker and Alpha-Blocker**
labetolol *(Normodyne, Trandate)*

*Side effects:* dizziness, weakness, drowsiness or fatigue, cold hands and feet, headache, upset stomach, diarrhea, constipation, dry mouth, skin, or eyes.

**Angiotensin-Converting Enzyme (ACE) Inhibitors**
benazepril *(Lotensin)*
captopril *(Capoten)*
enalapril *(Vasotec)*
fosinopril *(Monopril)*
lisinopril *(Prinivil, Zestril)*
quinapril *(Accupril)*
ramipril *(Altace)*
trandolapril *(Mavik)*

*Side effects:* dry cough, increased blood-potassium level, fatigue, dizziness, headaches, loss of taste.

**Angiotensin Receptor Blockers (ARBs)**
azilsartan *(Edarbi)*
candesartan *(Atacand)*
irbesartan *(Avapro)*
losartan *(Cozaar)*
olmesartan *(Benicar)*
telmisartan *(Micardis)*
valsartan *(Diovan)*

*Side effects:* dizziness, headache, drowsiness, nausea, vomiting, diarrhea, cough, elevated potassium levels.

## Diuretics

bumetanide *(Bumex)*
chlorthalidone *(Hygroton)*
eplerenone *(Inspra)**
furosemide *(Lasix)*
hydrochlorthiazide *(HCTZ, Hydodiuril)*
indapamide *(Lozol)*
metolazone *(Zaroxolyn)*
spironolactone *(Aldacone)**
triamterene *(Dyrenium)**
torsemide *(Demadex)*

*Side effects:* low potassium in the blood, too much potassium in the blood, low sodium levels, headache, dizziness, thirst, increased blood sugar, muscle cramps. *Denotes the diuretics that increase potassium.

## Calcium Channel Blockers

amlodipine *(Norvasc)*
diltiazem hydrochloride *(Cardizem, Cartia XT, Dilacor)*
felodipine *(Plendil)*
nicardipine *(Cardene)*
nifedipine *(Adalat, Procardia)*
nimodipine *(Nimotop)*
verapamil *(Calan, Covera, Isoptin, Verelan)*

*Side effects:* headache, constipation, rash, nausea, flushing, edema (fluid accumulation in tissues), drowsiness, low blood pressure.

## Vasodilators

hydralazine *(Apresoline)*
minoxidil *(Loniten)*

*Side effects:* chest pain, heart palpitations (fluttering or pounding heartbeat), rapid heartbeat, fluid retention, nausea or vomiting, dizziness, headache, flushing.

## Nerve Inhibitors

alpha-methyldopa *(Aldomet)*
clonidine *(Catapres)*

**Nerve Inhibitors (Continued)**
*Side effects:* fatigue, drowsiness or sedation, dizziness with change in position, impotence, constipation, abnormally slow heart rate, dry mouth, headache

## Blood Thinners

**Antiplatelet agents**
abciximab *(ReoPro)* IV only
aspirin
cangrelor *(Kengreal)* IV only
clopidogrel *(Plavix)*
eptifibatide *(Integrilin)* IV only
prasugrel *(Effient)*
ticagrelor *(Brilinta)*
tirofiban *(Aggrastat)* IV only
*Side effects:* nausea, upset stomach, stomach pain, diarrhea, rash, itching, major and minor bleeding.

**Anticoagulants**
apixiaban *(Eliquis)*
bivalirudin *(Angiomax)* Injection only
dabigatran *(Pradaxa)*
dalteparin *(Fragmin)* Injection only
enoxaparin *(Lovenox)* Injection only
edoxaban (Savaysa)
fondaparinux *(Arixtra)* Injection only
heparin *(Heparin)** Injection only
warfarin *(Coumadin)*
*Side effects:* passing blood in urine or feces, bruising, prolonged nosebleeds (lasting longer than ten minutes), bleeding gums, vomiting blood or coughing up blood, sudden severe back pain, major or minor bleeding, difficulty breathing or chest pain.

**Thrombolytics**
tPA or tissue Plasminogen Activator *(Alteplase, Activase)* IV only
reteplase *(Retavase)* IV only

tenecteplase *(TNKase)* IV only
streptokinase *(Kabikinase, Streptase)* IV only
**Thrombolytics (Continued)**

*Side effects:* serious internal bleeding, bruising or bleeding at the access site, damage to the blood vessel, migration of a blood clot to another part of vascular system.

## Drugs for Angina (Chest pain)

**Nitrates**

Nitrates, beta-blockers, calcium channel blockers and ranolazine (Ranexa) for chronic stable angina (*See* pages 112–114), are used to treat angina.

isosorbide dinitrate *(Sorbitrate, Dilatrate, Isordil)*
isosorbide mononitrate *(ISMO, Monoket, Imdur)*
nitroglycerine ointment *(nitroglycerine ointment), (Nitro-Bid)*
nitroglycerine patch *(Transderm-Nitro, Nitro-Dur, Mini tran)*
nitroglycerine spray *(NitroMist)*
nitroglycerine tablet *(Nitrostat)*
oral nitroglycerine *(nitroglycerine ER), Nitro-Time*

*Side effects:* headeaches, dizziness, lightheadedness, nausea, constipation, abdominal pain, or dry mouth.

# Body Mass Index (BMI) Table

| Height (inches) | Normal | | | | | | Overweight | | | | | Obese | | | | | | | | | | Extreme Obesity | | | | | | | | | | | | | | |
|---|---|---|---|---|---|---|---|---|---|---|---|---|---|---|---|---|---|---|---|---|---|---|---|---|---|---|---|---|---|---|---|---|---|---|---|---|
| BMI | 19 | 20 | 21 | 22 | 23 | 24 | 25 | 26 | 27 | 28 | 29 | 30 | 31 | 32 | 33 | 34 | 35 | 36 | 37 | 38 | 39 | 40 | 41 | 42 | 43 | 44 | 45 | 46 | 47 | 48 | 49 | 50 | 51 | 52 | 53 | 54 |
| | | | | | | | | | | | | | | | Body Weight (pounds) | | | | | | | | | | | | | | | | | | | | | |
| 58 | 91 | 96 | 100 | 105 | 110 | 115 | 119 | 124 | 129 | 134 | 138 | 143 | 148 | 153 | 158 | 162 | 167 | 172 | 177 | 181 | 186 | 191 | 196 | 201 | 205 | 210 | 215 | 220 | 224 | 229 | 234 | 239 | 244 | 248 | 253 | 258 |
| 59 | 94 | 99 | 104 | 109 | 114 | 119 | 124 | 128 | 133 | 138 | 143 | 148 | 153 | 158 | 163 | 168 | 173 | 178 | 183 | 188 | 193 | 198 | 203 | 208 | 212 | 217 | 222 | 227 | 232 | 237 | 242 | 247 | 252 | 257 | 262 | 267 |
| 60 | 97 | 102 | 107 | 112 | 118 | 123 | 128 | 133 | 138 | 143 | 148 | 153 | 158 | 163 | 168 | 174 | 179 | 184 | 189 | 194 | 199 | 204 | 209 | 215 | 220 | 225 | 230 | 235 | 240 | 245 | 250 | 255 | 261 | 266 | 271 | 276 |
| 61 | 100 | 106 | 111 | 116 | 122 | 127 | 132 | 137 | 143 | 148 | 153 | 158 | 164 | 169 | 174 | 180 | 185 | 190 | 195 | 201 | 206 | 211 | 217 | 222 | 227 | 232 | 238 | 243 | 248 | 254 | 259 | 264 | 269 | 275 | 280 | 285 |
| 62 | 104 | 109 | 115 | 120 | 126 | 131 | 136 | 142 | 147 | 153 | 158 | 164 | 169 | 175 | 180 | 186 | 191 | 196 | 202 | 207 | 213 | 218 | 224 | 229 | 235 | 240 | 246 | 251 | 256 | 262 | 267 | 273 | 278 | 284 | 289 | 295 |
| 63 | 107 | 113 | 118 | 124 | 130 | 135 | 141 | 146 | 152 | 158 | 163 | 169 | 175 | 180 | 186 | 191 | 197 | 203 | 208 | 214 | 220 | 225 | 231 | 237 | 242 | 248 | 254 | 259 | 265 | 270 | 278 | 282 | 287 | 293 | 299 | 304 |
| 64 | 110 | 116 | 122 | 128 | 134 | 140 | 145 | 151 | 157 | 163 | 169 | 174 | 180 | 186 | 192 | 197 | 204 | 209 | 215 | 221 | 227 | 232 | 238 | 244 | 250 | 256 | 262 | 267 | 273 | 279 | 285 | 291 | 296 | 302 | 308 | 314 |
| 65 | 114 | 120 | 126 | 132 | 138 | 144 | 150 | 156 | 162 | 168 | 174 | 180 | 186 | 192 | 198 | 204 | 210 | 216 | 222 | 228 | 234 | 240 | 246 | 252 | 258 | 264 | 270 | 276 | 282 | 288 | 294 | 300 | 306 | 312 | 318 | 324 |
| 66 | 118 | 124 | 130 | 136 | 142 | 148 | 155 | 161 | 167 | 173 | 179 | 186 | 192 | 198 | 204 | 210 | 216 | 223 | 229 | 235 | 241 | 247 | 253 | 260 | 266 | 272 | 278 | 284 | 291 | 297 | 303 | 309 | 315 | 322 | 328 | 334 |
| 67 | 121 | 127 | 134 | 140 | 146 | 153 | 159 | 166 | 172 | 178 | 185 | 191 | 198 | 204 | 211 | 217 | 223 | 230 | 236 | 242 | 249 | 255 | 261 | 268 | 274 | 280 | 287 | 293 | 299 | 306 | 312 | 319 | 325 | 331 | 338 | 344 |
| 68 | 125 | 131 | 138 | 144 | 151 | 158 | 164 | 171 | 177 | 184 | 190 | 197 | 203 | 210 | 216 | 223 | 230 | 236 | 243 | 249 | 256 | 262 | 269 | 276 | 282 | 289 | 295 | 302 | 308 | 315 | 322 | 328 | 335 | 341 | 348 | 354 |
| 69 | 128 | 135 | 142 | 149 | 155 | 162 | 169 | 176 | 182 | 189 | 196 | 203 | 209 | 216 | 223 | 230 | 236 | 243 | 250 | 257 | 263 | 270 | 277 | 284 | 291 | 297 | 304 | 311 | 318 | 324 | 331 | 338 | 345 | 351 | 358 | 365 |
| 70 | 132 | 139 | 146 | 153 | 160 | 167 | 174 | 181 | 188 | 195 | 202 | 209 | 216 | 222 | 229 | 236 | 243 | 250 | 257 | 264 | 271 | 278 | 285 | 292 | 299 | 306 | 313 | 320 | 327 | 334 | 341 | 348 | 355 | 362 | 369 | 376 |
| 71 | 136 | 143 | 150 | 157 | 165 | 172 | 179 | 186 | 193 | 200 | 208 | 215 | 222 | 229 | 236 | 243 | 250 | 257 | 265 | 272 | 279 | 286 | 293 | 301 | 308 | 315 | 322 | 329 | 338 | 343 | 351 | 358 | 365 | 372 | 379 | 386 |
| 72 | 140 | 147 | 154 | 162 | 169 | 177 | 184 | 191 | 199 | 206 | 213 | 221 | 228 | 235 | 242 | 250 | 258 | 265 | 272 | 279 | 287 | 294 | 302 | 309 | 316 | 324 | 331 | 338 | 346 | 353 | 361 | 368 | 375 | 383 | 390 | 397 |
| 73 | 144 | 151 | 159 | 166 | 174 | 182 | 189 | 197 | 204 | 212 | 219 | 227 | 235 | 242 | 250 | 257 | 265 | 272 | 280 | 288 | 295 | 302 | 310 | 318 | 325 | 333 | 340 | 348 | 355 | 363 | 371 | 378 | 386 | 393 | 401 | 408 |
| 74 | 148 | 155 | 163 | 171 | 179 | 186 | 194 | 202 | 210 | 218 | 225 | 233 | 241 | 249 | 256 | 264 | 272 | 280 | 287 | 295 | 303 | 311 | 319 | 326 | 334 | 342 | 350 | 358 | 365 | 373 | 381 | 389 | 396 | 404 | 412 | 420 |
| 75 | 152 | 160 | 168 | 176 | 184 | 192 | 200 | 208 | 216 | 224 | 232 | 240 | 248 | 256 | 264 | 272 | 279 | 287 | 295 | 303 | 311 | 319 | 327 | 335 | 343 | 351 | 359 | 367 | 375 | 383 | 391 | 399 | 407 | 415 | 423 | 431 |
| 76 | 156 | 164 | 172 | 180 | 189 | 197 | 205 | 213 | 221 | 230 | 238 | 246 | 254 | 263 | 271 | 279 | 287 | 295 | 304 | 312 | 320 | 328 | 336 | 344 | 353 | 361 | 369 | 377 | 385 | 394 | 402 | 410 | 418 | 426 | 435 | 443 |

Source: Adapted from *Clinical Guidelines on the Identification, Evaluation, and Treatment of Overweight and Obesity in Adults: The Evidence Report.*

# Resources

**Adult Congenital Heart Association (ACHA)**
3300 Henry Avenue, Suite 112
Philadelphia, PA 19119
Phone: (888) 921-ACHA
www.achaheart.org

**American Heart Association**
National Center
7272 Grandville Avenue
Dallas, TX 75231
Phone: (800) AHA-USA1 (242-8721)
www.heart.org

**American Society of Nuclear Cardiology (ASNC)**
4340 East-West Highway, Suite 1120
Bethesda, MD 20814
Phone: (301) 215-7575
www.asnc.org

**Heart Failure Society of America, Inc.**
9211 Corporate Boulevard, Suite 270
Rockville, MD 20850
Phone: (301) 312-8635
www.hfsa.org

**National Heart, Lung, and Blood Institute (NHLBI)**
Building 21
31 Center Drive
Bethesda, MD 20892
Phone: (301) 592-8573
www.nhlbi.nih.gov

**National Institute of Neurological Disorders and Stroke (NINDS)**
P.O. Box 5801
Bethesda, MD 20824
Phone: (800) 352-9424
www.ninds.nih.gov

**NIH Neurological Institute**
P.O. Box 5801
Bethesda, MD 20824
Phone: (800) 352-9424
www.ninds.nih.gov

**Pulmonary Hypertension Association**
801 Roeder Road, Suite 1000
Silver Spring, MD 20910
Phone: (800) 748-7274
www.phassociation.org

**The Mended Hearts, Inc.**
8150 North Central Expressway, M2248
Dallas, TX 75206
Phone: (888) 432-7899
www.mendedhearts.org

# GLOSSARY

## A

**ACE inhibitors (ACEs):** Also called *angiotensin-converting enzyme inhibitors*, ACEs belong to a class of drugs used to lower high blood pressure and treat patients with heart failure and after heart attacks. ACEs block the formation of the chemical that causes tiny arteries to constrict.

**alpha-blockers:** Blood pressure-lowering drugs that block the stimulation of specialized nerves.

**angina:** The medical term is angina pectoris. Angina is chest pressure and pain caused when the heart doesn't receive enough oxygen.

**AngioJet:** A high-pressure spray device used with a catheter to break up blood clots.

**angioplasty:** Also called *balloon angioplasty* or *percutaneous transluminal coronary angioplasty (PTCA)*, angioplasty is an invasive procedure that treats the inside of coronary arteries without opening the chest.

**angiotensin:** A chemical the body produces that causes small arteries *(arterioles)* to constrict.

**antiarrhythrnics:** Medications that correct heart rhythm problems.

**anticoagulants:** Blood-thinning drugs that inhibit special proteins that form blood clots.

**antiplatelets:** Drugs that reduce the ability of the blood to clot by inhibiting the normal function of platelets (blood clotting cells).

**aorta:** The large artery that receives blood from the heart's left ventricle and carries it to the body.

121

**apoproteins:** Proteins the body uses to coat cholesterol so that it can be transported in the blood.

**ARBs (angiotensin receptor blockers):** Drugs prescribed for high blood pressure and to treat heart failure. They block the chemical that causes tiny arteries to constrict.

**arrhythmia:** Abnormal heartbeat.

**arterioles:** Tiny arteries, the blood vessels that carry blood, oxygen, and nutrients to cells in the body.

**arteriosclerosis:** Commonly called "hardening of the arteries," arteriosclerosis is a process in which the arteries become thicker and harder, losing their natural elasticity.

**artery:** A blood vessel that carries blood away from the heart.

**atherosclerosis:** A process in which deposits of cholesterol, cellular waste products, calcium, and other substances build up in the inner lining of arteries.

**atriums (or atria):** Top chambers of the heart.

**B**

**balloon angioplasty:** *See* angioplasty

**beta-blockers:** A class of drugs often used to alleviate angina and treat high blood pressure. They block adrenaline's effect on the heart, decreasing heart rate, reducing the strength of the heart's contractions, and lowering blood pressure.

**blood pressure:** A measurement of the force when the heart pumps blood into the arteries and out to the body, and the force of the arteries as they resist the blood from the heart. It's expressed in millimeters of mercury (mmHg).

**brachytherapy:** Also called *intracoronary radiation,* brachytherapy involves exposing the arteries to gamma or beta radiation to reduce the incidence of arterial renarrowing.

**bruits:** The rough, turbulent sounds of blood moving through narrowed arteries. Doctors use a stethoscope on the neck, abdomen, and elsewhere to detect bruits (French for noise).

**C**

**calcium channel blockers:** Drugs that block or inhibit the movement of calcium in the heart, nerves, and blood vessel walls. These drugs reduce blood pressure and dilate coronary arteries.

**capillaries:** Very small vessels, often too small to see, that connect the arterial and venous blood systems.

**cardiac angiography:** Also called *arteriography, angiocardiography,* or *cardiac catheterization and angiography,* this invasive diagnostic technique uses flexible tubes called *catheters* threaded through the arteries. It can show blood flow problems and blockages in the coronary arteries.

**cardiac positron-emission tomography (PET):** A nuclear imaging technology that can measure blood flow and metabolism in the heart.

**catheter:** A long, slender, flexible tube used in angiography that is threaded through the arteries.

**CT or CAT scan (computed tomography scan):** An imaging technique in which an X-ray beam is passed through the body as the scanner is rapidly rotated around the body. It produces a detailed cross-section of the body.

**cholesterol:** A waxy, fatlike substance that is found in every cell in the body. It is used to help digest fats, strengthen cell membranes, and make some types of hormones and vitamins. It is also a major component of plaque.

**coronary arteries:** The arteries that branch from the aorta, divide into smaller arteries, and provide blood for the heart muscle.

**coronary artery bypass graft surgery (CABG):** Surgery in which pieces of blood vessels are stitched around blocked arteries, creating bypasses around blockages. Often called "cabbage."

**coronary heart disease (CHD):** Also called *coronary artery disease (CAD)* or *ischemic heart disease,* it is a condition caused when arteries become narrowed by plaque.

**coronary occlusion:** Blockage of a coronary artery that restricts the blood supply.

**coronary thrombosis:** Another name for coronary occlusion, a heart attack caused by a clot blocking blood supply to the heart.

**cyanotic:** Skin that is bluish in color, which may be a sign of vascular disease or lack of oxygen.

# D

**diabetes:** Called *diabetes mellitus,* it's a disease in which the body isn't able to produce and/or respond to the hormone insulin, which converts blood sugar into energy.

**dissection of the aorta:** A life-threatening condition in which the inner lining of the major artery that leads away from the heart (aorta) becomes torn and may cause severe chest pain.

**diuretics:** Drugs that flush excess water and sodium from the body by increasing urination.

**Doppler ultrasound:** Part of an echocardiogram study that produces heart sounds and displays a picture of the blood flowing between the chambers of the heart, and measures internal pressures.

# E

**echocardiogram:** A diagnostic test in which sound waves are used to "bounce back" images of the heart.

**electrocardiography (ECG):** A diagnostic test that records the electrical activity of the heart.

**electron beam computed tomography (EBCT):** This ultrafast CT scan detects CHD by measuring calcium in the blood vessels.

**endotracheal tube:** A breathing tube used during bypass surgery.

**estrogen:** A female hormone. Oral contraceptives and hormone replacement therapy (HRT) use synthetic forms of estrogen.

**exercise ECG:** Also called a *stress ECG* or *treadmill test,* it's a diagnostic test that records the electrical activity of the heart under stress *(exercise or medication).*

# F

**fibrates:** Triglyceride-lowering medications.

**fish oils:** Obtained from eating fish or by taking supplements. Two of the most important omega-3 fatty acids contained in fish oil are *eicosapentaenoic acid (EPA)* and *docosahexaenoic acid (DHA).* Fish oil is FDA approved to lower triglycerides levels.

# G

**gene therapy:** A new technology for treating disease, gene therapy involves introducing genetic material into cells to cause certain actions.

# H

**heart attack:** Also called *myocardial infarction,* a heart attack occurs when the blood supply to a portion of the heart muscle is blocked and the part of the heart that doesn't receive blood becomes damaged and dies.

**heart failure:** A condition in which the heart becomes unable to pump efficiently and supply the body with the blood it needs.

**high blood pressure:** Also called *hypertension,* high blood pressure occurs when the blood pressure is 130/80 mmHg or higher, which strains the heart.

**high-density lipoprotein:** So-called "good" cholesterol, HDL cholesterol contains mostly protein. When there's excess cholesterol in the blood, HDL cholesterol picks up cholesterol deposited in the arteries and transports it to the liver for disposal.

**Holter monitoring:** Also called *ambulatory ECG monitoring,* it's a variation of electrocardiography that monitors and records the heart's electrical activity during everyday activities. It's used to detect heart problems that come and go.

**homocysteine:** An amino acid that's a by-product of the body's use of protein. High levels of homocysteine have been associated with a low intake of folate, vitamin B6, and vitamin B12 and is associated with heart disease.

**hydrogenation:** A process used in making margarine and shortening in which unsaturated fats become more highly saturated fats.

# I

**in-stent restenosis:** A condition in which arteries that are treated with stents (fine-mesh tubes) become renarrowed.

**insulin:** A hormone produced by the pancreas that helps the body convert blood sugar *(glucose)* into a usable form for energy.

**internal mammary arteries (IMAs):** Two arteries located on the inside chest wall that are often used in bypass surgery.

**intracoronary radiation:** Also called *brachytherapy,* it's a procedure in which arteries treated with stents are exposed to radiation in an effort to stop or slow down the formation of scar tissue.

**intravascular ultrasound (IVUS):** An imaging technology in which a small device mounted on the tip of a catheter is inserted into coronary arteries. The device sends back images of the inside of the arteries using ultrasound technology.

**ischemia:** Reduced blood flow to an organ. In most cases, this reduction is caused by a blockage or narrowing of an artery.

**ischemic heart disease:** Another name for coronary artery disease or coronary heart disease. Ischemic heart disease is caused by arteries becoming narrowed and causing a reduced blood supply to the heart.

**L**

**lipoprotein profile:** A fasting blood test that measures total cholesterol, HDL and LDL cholesterol, and triglyceride levels. All adults should have a lipoprotein profile performed at least once every five years.

**lipoproteins:** The protein "packages" that transport cholesterol in the blood.

**low-density lipoprotein:** So-called "bad" cholesterol, LDL cholesterol contributes to plaque building in the arteries.

**M**

**magnetic resonance imaging (MRI):** Diagnostic test that uses powerful magnets and radio waves to produce images of the inside of the body.

**myocardial infarction (MI):** The medical term for heart attack. When blood supply to a part of the heart is severely reduced or blocked, a heart attack can occur. The area of the heart muscle on the other side of the blockage begins to die and results in permanent damage to the heart. *See also* heart attack.

**N**

**nerve inhibitors:** Drugs used to reduce blood pressure by affecting control centers in the brain that keep these nerves from narrowing (constricting) blood vessels.

**niacin B:** Vitamin that can lower tryglycerides and increase HDL cholesterol.

**nitrate:** A type of anti-anginal medication used to widen the coronary arteries.

**nuclear scanning:** A variety of diagnostic tests that involve injecting a tiny amount of radioactive material into the bloodstream and taking images of the radiation given off by the material.

**O**

**orbital atherectomy:** A diamond-coated burr used for calicified coronary lesions.

**P**

**PCSK9 inhibitors:** Medication injected once or twice monthly to reduce LDL cholesertols.

**percutaneous transluminal coronary angioplasty (PTCA):** *See angioplasty.*

**pericarditis:** Inflammation of the fibrous sac that surrounds the heart *(pericardium).* The chest pain caused by pericarditis can mimic angina.

**Prinzmetal's angina:** *See* variant angina.

**plaque:** A mixture of fatty substances, cholesterol, cellular waste products, calcium, and other substances that become deposited in the inner lining of arteries.

**platelets:** The clotting cells in blood.

**pressure wire:** A diagnostic tool used in the cath lab that measures pressures inside arteries to determine the significance of a narrowing.

**progestin:** A synthetic form of the female hormone progesterone. Progestin is often used in birth control pills and hormone replacement therapy (HRT).

**pulmonary embolism:** Blood clot in the lung.

**pump oxygenator:** Commonly called a *heart-lung machine,* it's used to keep the blood flowing and oxygenated while the heart is stopped during surgery.

**R**

**reperfusion therapy:** A variety of techniques (including medications, angioplasty, and surgery) that may be used to restore blood flow to areas of the heart damaged by a heart attack.

**resins:** Cholesterol-lowering drugs that cause the intestines to absorb less cholesterol from the digestive tract.

**restenosis:** The term used when arteries become narrowed again following a procedure to open them.

**risk factors:** Traits or lifestyle habits that put one at greater risk for developing certain illnesses or conditions.

**rotational atherectomy:** A procedure in which the cardiologist uses a diamond-coated burr to treat conditions such as calcified plaque.

**S**

**saphenous vein:** The vein that lies just inside the leg. It's often used in bypass surgery.

**saturated fat:** The type of fat that comes from animal sources (meat, poultry, fish, egg yolks, dairy products). Solid at room temperature, saturated fat has been associated with the plaque building of atherosclerosis.

**silent ischemia:** A temporary shortage of blood and oxygen to the heart that doesn't produce any symptoms.

**single photon emission computed tomography (SPECT):** One of the most commonly used nuclear imaging technologies. It involves injecting a radioactive material and then taking images of the chest.

**statins:** Drugs often used to reduce cholesterol, statins work directly on the liver to block the manufacture of cholesterol.

**stenosis:** Narrowing. In the case of CHD, narrowing of blood vessels.

**stents:** Small, fine-mesh tubes that are inserted into arteries to keep them open.

**stroke:** Also called a "brain attack," a stroke occurs when one or more blood vessels supplying the brain become blocked, causing the death of brain cells.

**sudden cardiac death (SCD):** Sudden and unexpected death caused by the total loss of heart function in someone with or without diagnosed heart disease.

**T**

**tachycardia:** Abnormally rapid heartbeat.

**thrombolytics:** Clot-busting drugs used in the treatment of heart attack.

**total blood cholesterol:** A combination of low-density lipoprotein (LDL) and high-density lipoprotein (HDL) cholesterol and triglycerides.

**transmyocardial revascularization (TMR):** A technique in which the surgeon drills laser holes into the heart's pumping chamber to relieve chest pain.

**triglycerides:** A type of blood fat. Elevated levels of triglycerides are associated with CHD.

**V**

**variant angina:** Also called *Prinzmetal's angina,* it's a less common type of chest pain caused when the muscle fibers surrounding the coronary arteries spasm and narrow or completely close off blood vessels that feed the heart.

**vasodilators:** Medications that reduce blood pressure by dilating blood vessels.

**vein:** One of many vessels that carry blood to the heart.

**ventricles:** The lower chambers *(one right and one left)* of the heart.

**venules:** Small veins.

**very low-density lipoprotein (VLDL):** A type of cholesterol-protein package that contains cholesterol, triglycerides, and protein.

# INDEX

131

# ABOUT THE AUTHOR

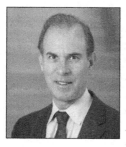 **Barry M. Cohen, M.D.,** is the medical director of the Cardiac Catherization Laboratory and co-director of the Valve and Structural Heart Program at the Morristown Medical Center's Gagnon Cardiovascular Institute in New Jersey. He is a practicing clinical cardiologist with the Atlantic Medical Group's Associates in Cardiovascular Disease in Springfield, New Jersey.

A native of Montreal, Dr. Cohen completed his undergraduate studies at McGill University and received his medical degree from the University of Sherbrooke in Canada. Following his clinical cardiology fellowship at the Mount Sinai Medical Center in New York City, he completed an interventional cardiology fellowship at the University of California–San Diego Medical Center.

Dr. Cohen is a diplomate of the American Boards of Interventional Cardiology, Cardiovascular Diseases and Internal Medicine. He is a fellow of the American College of Cardiology, the Society for Cardiovascular Angiography and Interventions, and the Royal College of Physicians and Surgeons of Canada. He is past president of the New Jersey Society of Interventional Cardiology. Dr. Cohen is an associate clinical professor of medicine at Mount Sinai's Icahn School of Medicine and at Thomas Jefferson's Sidney Kimmel Medical College.

Dr. Cohen has published numerous scientific papers and abstracts in interventional cardiology. He has pioneered rotational atherectomy, used in the treatment of complex calcified coronary arterial blockages. He has been an investigator test-

145

ing new stent designs and Impella-assisted high-risk percutaneous coronary intervention (PCI). Dr. Cohen was the first physician in New Jersey to use the Arctic Sun "Cold Suit" to preserve brain function in a patient after cardiac arrest. He treats stroke patients who have associated heart defects. Dr. Cohen is a leading clinical investigator at Gagnon, treating patients with valvular heart disease. The medical center's team is one of the busiest valve teams in the country both in mitral and aortic valve (transcatheter aortic valve replacement, or TAVR) procedures.

## Consumer Health Titles from Addicus Books

Visit our online catalog at www.AddicusBooks.com

## To Order Books:
**Visit us online at:** www.AddicusBooks.com
**Call toll free:** (800) 888-4741

For discounts on bulk purchases, call our Special Sales
Department at (402) 330-7493.
Or email us at: info@Addicus Books.com

Addicus Books
P. O. Box 45327
Omaha, NE 68145

*Addicus Books is dedicated to publishing consumer health books
that comfort and educate.*

Made in the USA
Middletown, DE
24 October 2020